food & diet counter

Complete nutritional facts for every diet!

Dr. Wynnie Chan hamlyn

First published in Great Britain in 2003 by Hamlyn,
a division of Octopus Publishing Group Ltd,
2–4 Heron Quays, London E14 4JP

copyright © Octopus Publishing Group Ltd 2003

Distributed in the United States and Canada by
Sterling Publishing Co., Inc.
387 Park Avenue South, New York, NY 10016-8810

ISBN 0 600 60888 3

A CIP catalogue record for this book is available
from the British Library

Printed and bound in China

10 9 8 7 6 5 4 3 2 1

Nutrient information has been calculated using data from the
UK Food Nutrient Databank which is available from The Food
Standards Agency (FSA). Some values have been estimated
based on similar foods.
The information in this book is intended only as a guide to
following a healthy diet. People with special dietary
requirements of any kind should consult appropriate medical
professionals before changing their diet.

CONTENTS

Whether you want to lose just a few pounds or rather more, eating healthily is vital. This does not mean cutting out all of your favorite treats completely, just eating them in moderation. If you're not enjoying your food, you are less likely to stick to your diet and exercise regime.

Losing weight doesn't just mean that you'll have more energy and feel better about yourself, it also decreases the risk of developing various ailments, including diabetes, hypertension, coronary heart disease, stroke, respiratory problems, gallstones and some cancers.

What is a healthy weight?

The formula used to establish whether a person is too thin, the right weight, fat or obese is called the Body Mass Index (BMI). This is a simple measurement of weight against height, and can be calculated using the following equation:

$$\frac{\text{weight (kg)}}{\text{height (m)} \times \text{height (m)}}$$

So, a person weighing 56kg who is 1.5m tall has a BMI of 25:
56 ÷ (1.5 x 1.5) = 25.
Alternatively:

$$\frac{\text{weight (lbs.)} \times 703}{\text{height (in.)} \times \text{height (in.)}}$$

So, the same person, weighing 123lbs. who is 59 in. tall has the same BMI of 25:
123 x 703 ÷ (59 x 59) = 25.

BMI RATINGS

below 20:	underweight
20–24.9:	normal weight
25–29.9:	overweight
30–39.9:	moderate obesity
Over 40:	severe obesity

Balanced diets

Including foods from the five food groups means that you are meeting your requirements for nutrients.

THE FIVE GROUPS ARE:

1 Bread, cereals and potatoes. This group is rich in starchy carbohydrates and includes breakfast cereals, rice, pasta, noodles, yams and oats and should form the basis of most meals. Foods in this group are rich in insoluble fiber, calcium, iron and B vitamins, which are needed to keep your bowels, bones and blood healthy. Try to eat wholegrain, wholewheat or high-fiber versions of breads and cereals.

2 Fruits and vegetables.

These are important sources of antioxidants such as vitamin C and beta-carotene (vegetable vitamin A), which protect us from cancers and heart disease. They are also rich in soluble fiber, which helps lower blood cholesterol. Try to include five portions of different fruits and vegetables in your diet each day, whether fresh, frozen, canned, dried or juiced.

A portion of fruit equals:
■ 1 slice of pineapple, grapefruit, melon or watermelon, or half a mango or papaya
■ 1 whole apple, avocado, banana, orange, peach or pear
■ 2 small apricots, clementines, figs, kiwi fruit, passion fruit, plums, satsumas or tomatoes
■ 1 cupful of berries, cherries or grapes
■ $1/2$ cup stewed apples or applesauce, apricots, fruit cocktail, pears, peaches or pineapple, or fresh fruit salad
■ $1/4$ cup dried apricots, bananas, cranberries, dates, figs, papaya, pineapple or raisins
■ 1 (8fl. oz) glass of fruit juice (not fruit drinks)

A portion of vegetables equals:
■ $1/2$ cup broccoli, brussels sprouts, cabbage, cauliflower, radishes, turnip, rutabaga, chard, winter greens, kale, pak choi, arugula, romaine lettuce, spinach, eggplant, carrots, green beans, mushrooms, onions, peas, peppers or squash
■ half a cupful of alfalfa, baked beans, beansprouts, sprouting broccoli, black beans, chickpeas, kidney beans, lentils or soy beans
■ 4 oz of salad
■ 1 (8fl. oz) glass of carrot, beetroot or wheatgrass juice

3 Milk and dairy foods.

These are excellent sources of calcium, protein and vitamins A and B12, which are essential for healthy bones, skin and blood. Include a couple of reduced-fat servings from this food group each day.

4 Meat, fish and alternatives.

The main nutrients supplied by this food group include iron, protein, B vitamins, zinc and magnesium, which help to maintain healthy blood and an efficient immune system. Choose at most two servings of lean red meat, fish, chicken, nuts, turkey, eggs, beans or pulses. The last two are great protein alternatives, as is tofu, which is also a good source of calcium.

5 Foods containing sugar or fat. Minimize your intake of savory snacks, cookies, cakes, chips, pastries, candy, chocolate, pies, butter and carbonated drinks, as these will hinder your efforts to lose weight.

Watch the fat

Gram for gram, fat has more than twice as many calories as protein and carbohydrates:

Calories per gram	cal	J
fat	9	37
protein	4	17
carbohydrate	3.75	16

Foods with high levels of fat tend to be low in fiber and are not filling, so we eat more of these than high-carbohydrate foods. This raises the calorie intake even farther. Most of us should eat at least 25g (1oz) less fat a day.

GOOD FAT, BAD FAT

All fats will increase your weight if you eat too much, but not all raise the risk of developing disease. There are three types of fat: saturated, monounsaturated and polyunsaturated. The former raise levels of "bad" cholesterol in the blood. Cholesterol is carried around the body by two proteins: low-density lipoprotein (LDL) and high-density lipoprotein (HDL). When levels of LDL cholesterol are raised in the blood, it may be deposited on blood vessel walls, narrowing them so they become blocked. As blood supply to the heart is interrupted it can lead to a heart attack which in severe cases can be fatal.

HDL is considered good as it carries cholesterol from various parts of the body to the liver where it can be disposed of.

As a general rule, fats that are hard at room temperature will contain the most saturated fat. Cakes, butter, cheese, cookies, cooking fats, pastries, pies, fatty meat, whole milk and hard margarine provide the most saturated fats in our diets so cut down on these.

The monounsaturated and polyunsaturated fats are found in vegetable oils and fat spreads, and are considered healthier than saturated fats. Replacing the latter with the other versions can lower levels of LDL cholesterol.

Fatty or oily fish like sardines, salmon, mackerel, herring and trout contain polyunsaturated fats called omega-3 fats. These help to protect against heart disease. We should eat a serving of oily fish each week.

Guideline Daily Amounts

Guideline Daily Amounts (GDAs) are daily guideline figures recommended by health professionals for intake of calories, fat and saturates for adult women and men. These are average figures and personal requirements will vary with age, weight and levels of activity.

AVERAGE DAILY REQUIREMENT

	women	men
cal	2000	2500
fat	70g	95g
saturates	20g	30g

Dietary Reference Values

Dietary Reference Values (DRVs) are daily recommendations that have been set by the Department of Health for the nutrients considered sufficient for most adults and children. The table below gives the average daily requirement for protein, carbohydrate and fiber. If you are trying to lose weight, you will need less, and should discuss the exact amounts with your doctor or dietician.

AVERAGE DAILY REQUIREMENT

	women	men
protein	46g	56g
carbohydrate	225g	300g
fibre	18g	18g

How to use this book
It lists the energy, as calories (cal) and joules (J), fat, saturated fat, protein, carbohydrate and fiber contained in more than 1500 foods. Nutrient values have been expressed as average servings so no calculator is needed.

The information shows where the energy comes from in any food so, if you're on a low-fat, low-carbohydrate diet or have any other special requirements, you can work out exactly how much you can have of any food.

Note
The average portion sizes of foods were obtained from *Food Portion Sizes, Second Edition,* HMSO, 1999. This information is based on a) weighed dietary surveys conducted by the Ministry of Agriculture, Fisheries and Food, b) information from manufacturers and c) by weighing numerous samples of foods such as takeout dishes.

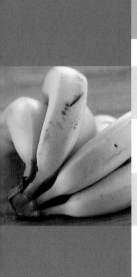

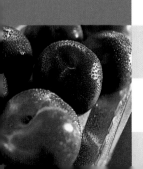

FRUITS	AVERAGE PORTION oz
Apples, cooking	4.5
Apples, cooking, stewed with sugar	3.8
Apples, cooking, stewed without sugar	3
Apples, Cox's Pippin	3.5
Apples, Golden Delicious	3.5
Apples, Granny Smith	3.5
Apples, red dessert	3.5
Apricots	2.8
Apricots, canned in juice	5
Apricots, dried	4.2
Apricots, stewed with sugar	5
Apricots, stewed without sugar	5
Avocado, Fuerte	6
Avocado, Hass	6
Banana chips	0.5
Bananas	3.5
Bilberries	40
Blackberries	3.5
Blackberries, stewed with sugar	5
Blackberries, stewed without sugar	5
Blackcurrants	3.5
Blackcurrants, canned in juice	5
Blackcurrants, canned in syrup	5
Blackcurrants, stewed with sugar	5
Blackcurrants, stewed without sugar	5
Cape gooseberry	2
Carambola	4.2
Cherries	2.8
Cherries, canned in syrup	2.4
Cherries, glacé	0.5
Clementines	2
Cranberries	2.6
Currants	0.8
Custard apples	2

Unless otherwise stated, fruits are prepared but uncooked.

ENERGY cal	ENERGY J	FAT g	SATURATED FAT g	PROTEIN g	CARBOHYDRATE g	FIBER g
46	196	Trace	Trace	0	12	2.1
81	345	Trace	Trace	0	21	1.3
28	117	Trace	Trace	0	7	1.3
46	195	Trace	Trace	1	11	2
43	185	Trace	Trace	0	11	1.7
45	193	Trace	Trace	0	12	1.7
51	217	Trace	Trace	0	13	1.9
25	107	Trace	Trace	1	6	1.4
48	206	Trace	Trace	1	12	1.3
190	809	1	Trace	5	44	7.6
101	431	Trace	Trace	1	26	2.2
38	161	Trace	Trace	1	9	2.1
327	1349	33	6.1	4	3	5.9
330	1362	34	8.1	3	3	5.9
66	278	4	Trace	0	8	0.2
95	403	1	0.1	1	23	1.1
12	51	Trace	Trace	0	3	0.7
25	104	Trace	Trace	1	5	3.1
78	335	Trace	Trace	1	19	3.4
29	123	Trace	Trace	1	6	3.6
28	121	Trace	Trace	1	7	3.6
43	189	Trace	Trace	1	11	4.3
101	428	Trace	Trace	1	26	3.6
81	353	Trace	Trace	1	21	3.9
34	144	Trace	Trace	1	8	4.3
32	131	Trace	Trace	1	7	1
38	163	1	0.1	1	9	1.6
38	162	Trace	Trace	1	9	0.7
48	207	Trace	Trace	0	13	0.4
39	159	Trace	Trace	0	9	0
22	95	Trace	Trace	1	5	0.7
11	49	Trace	Trace	0	3	2.3
67	285	Trace	Trace	1	17	0.5
41	178	Trace	Trace	1	10	1.4

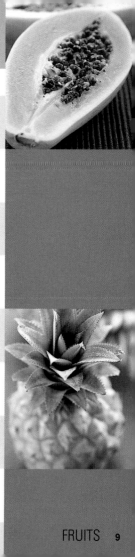

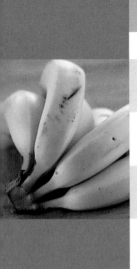

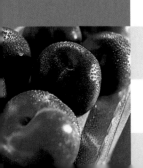

FRUITS	AVERAGE PORTION oz
Damsons	2.8
Damsons, stewed with sugar	3.5
Damsons, stewed without sugar	3.5
Dates	3.5
Dates, stoned and dried	2
Durian	2.8
Figs	1.9
Figs, dried	3
Fruit cocktail, canned in juice	4
Fruit cocktail, canned in syrup	4
Fruit salad, mixed	5
Golden raisins	0.6
Gooseberries	3.5
Gooseberries, canned in syrup	5
Gooseberries, stewed with sugar	5
Gooseberries, stewed without sugar	5
Grapefruit	8
Grapefruit, canned in juice	4.2
Grapefruit, canned in syrup	4.2
Grapes	3.5
Greengages	3.5
Greengages, stewed with sugar	3.5
Greengages, stewed without sugar	3.5
Guavas	3.5
Guavas, canned in syrup	4
Kiwi fruit	2
Kumquats	0.3
Kumquats, canned in syrup	0.3
Lemons, unpeeled	2
Limes, unpeeled	1.4
Loganberries, canned in juice	5
Loganberries, stewed with sugar	5
Loganberries, stewed without sugar	5
Lychees	3.2

Unless otherwise stated, fruits are prepared but uncooked.

ENERGY cal	ENERGY J	FAT g	SATURATED FAT g	PROTEIN g	CARBOHYDRATE g	FIBER g
30	130	Trace	Trace	0	8	1.4
74	316	Trace	Trace	0	19	1.5
34	147	Trace	Trace	1	9	1.6
124	530	Trace	Trace	2	31	1.8
162	691	1	0.1	2	41	2.4
109	460	1	Trace	2	23	3
24	102	1	0.1	1	5	0.8
176	747	1	Trace	3	41	5.8
33	140	Trace	Trace	0	8	1.2
66	281	Trace	Trace	0	17	1.2
77	332	Trace	Trace	1	19	2.1
50	211	Trace	Trace	0	12	0.4
40	170	1	0.1	1	9	2.4
102	434	Trace	Trace	1	26	2.4
76	321	Trace	Trace	1	18	2.7
22	92	Trace	Trace	1	4	2.8
69	291	Trace	Trace	2	16	3
36	144	Trace	Trace	1	9	0.5
72	308	Trace	Trace	1	19	0.7
60	257	Trace	Trace	0	15	0.7
41	173	Trace	Trace	1	10	2.1
81	347	Trace	Trace	1	21	1.9
36	155	Trace	Trace	1	9	1.9
26	112	1	Trace	1	5	3.7
68	292	Trace	Trace	0	18	3.4
29	124	Trace	Trace	1	6	1.1
3	15	Trace	Trace	0	1	0.3
11	46	Trace	Trace	0	3	0.1
8	36	1	0.1	0	1	1.7
4	14	0	0	0	0	1.1
141	601	Trace	Trace	1	37	2.2
70	300	Trace	Trace	1	18	2.8
20	87	Trace	Trace	1	4	2.9
52	223	Trace	Trace	1	13	0.6

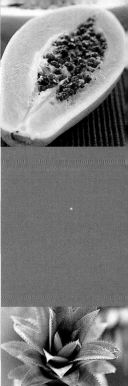

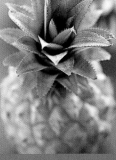

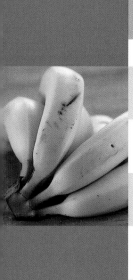

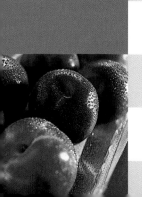

FRUITS	AVERAGE PORTION oz
Lychees, canned in syrup	2.8
Mandarin oranges, canned in juice	4
Mandarin oranges, canned in syrup	4.4
Mangoes	5.3
Mangoes, canned in syrup	3.7
Mangosteen	2
Melon, Canteloupe	5.3
Melon, Galia	5.3
Melon, Honeydew	7
Mixed candied peel	0.2
Nectarines	5.3
Oranges	5.6
Passion fruit	2
Paw-paw	5
Peaches	3.9
Peaches, canned in juice	4.2
Peaches, canned in syrup	4.2
Pears, canned in juice	4.7
Pears, canned in syrup	4.7
Pears, Comice	5.3
Pears, Conference	6
Pears, Nashi	5.3
Pears, William	5.3
Pineapple	2.8
Pineapple, canned in juice	1.4
Pineapple, canned in syrup	1.4
Plums, average, stewed with sugar	4.7
Plums, average, stewed without sugar	2.5
Plums, canned in syrup	2.8
Plums, Victoria	1.9
Plums, yellow	1.9
Pomegranate	1.9
Pomelo	2.8
Prickly pears	2.8

Unless otherwise stated, fruits are prepared but uncooked.

ENERGY cal	ENERGY J	FAT g	SATURATED FAT g	PROTEIN g	CARBOHYDRATE g	FIBER g
54	232	Trace	Trace	0	14	0.4
37	155	Trace	Trace	1	9	0.3
66	281	Trace	Trace	1	17	0.3
86	368	1	0.2	1	21	3.9
81	347	Trace	Trace	0	21	0.7
44	184	Trace	Trace	0	10	1
29	122	Trace	Trace	1	6	1.5
36	153	Trace	Trace	1	8	0.6
56	238	Trace	Trace	1	13	1.2
12	49	Trace	Trace	0	3	0.2
60	257	Trace	Trace	2	14	1.8
59	253	Trace	Trace	2	14	2.7
22	91	1	0.1	2	3	2
50	214	Trace	Trace	1	12	3.1
36	156	Trace	Trace	1	8	1.7
47	198	Trace	Trace	1	12	1
66	280	Trace	Trace	1	17	1.1
45	190	Trace	Trace	0	11	1.9
68	290	Trace	Trace	0	18	1.5
50	212	Trace	Trace	0	13	3
90	386	1	Trace	1	22	4.1
44	183	Trace	Trace	0	11	2.3
51	215	Trace	Trace	1	12	3.3
33	141	Trace	Trace	0	8	1
19	80	Trace	Trace	0	5	0.2
26	109	Trace	Trace	0	7	0.3
105	446	Trace	Trace	1	27	1.7
21	90	Trace	Trace	0	5	0.9
47	202	Trace	Trace	0	12	0.6
21	92	Trace	Trace	0	5	1
14	59	Trace	Trace	0	3	0.6
28	120	Trace	Trace	1	6	1.9
24	101	Trace	Trace	0	5	0.8
29	124	1	0.1	0	7	2.2

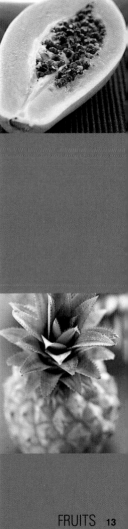

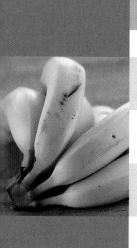

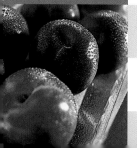

FRUITS	AVERAGE PORTION oz
Prunes, canned in juice	0.8
Prunes, canned in syrup	0.8
Prunes, dried	2.3
Prunes, stewed with sugar	0.8
Prunes, stewed without sugar	0.8
Quinces	3.2
Raisins	1
Rambutan	2.8
Raspberries	2
Raspberries, canned in syrup	3.2
Raspberries, stewed with sugar	3.2
Raspberries, stewed without sugar	3.2
Redcurrants	0.1
Redcurrants, stewed with sugar	5
Redcurrants, stewed without sugar	5
Rhubarb, canned in syrup	5
Rhubarb, stewed with sugar	5
Rhubarb, stewed without sugar	5
Satsumas	2.5
Sharon fruit	3.9
Starfruit	4.2
Strawberries	3.5
Sugar apples	2
Tangerines	2.5
Watermelon	7

Unless otherwise stated, fruits are prepared but uncooked.

ENERGY cal	ENERGY J	FAT g	SATURATED FAT g	PROTEIN g	CARBOHYDRATE g	FIBER g
19	80	Trace	Trace	0	5	0.6
22	93	Trace	Trace	0	6	0.7
93	397	Trace	Trace	2	22	3.8
25	105	Trace	Trace	0	6	0.7
19	83	Trace	0	0	5	0.8
23	99	Trace	Trace	0	6	1.7
82	348	Trace	Trace	1	21	0.6
55	234	Trace	Trace	1	13	0.5
15	65	1	0.1	1	3	1.5
79	337	Trace	Trace	1	20	1.4
57	244	1	0.1	1	14	2
22	95	1	0.1	1	4	2.2
0	2	Trace	Trace	0	0	0.1
74	318	Trace	Trace	1	19	3.8
24	106	Trace	Trace	1	5	4.1
43	182	Trace	Trace	1	11	1.1
67	284	Trace	Trace	1	16	1.7
10	42	Trace	Trace	1	1	1.8
25	109	Trace	Trace	1	6	0.9
80	342	Trace	Trace	1	20	1.8
38	163	1	0.1	1	9	1.6
27	113	Trace	Trace	1	6	1.1
41	178	Trace	Trace	1	10	1.4
25	103	Trace	Trace	1	6	0.9
62	266	1	0.2	1	14	0.2

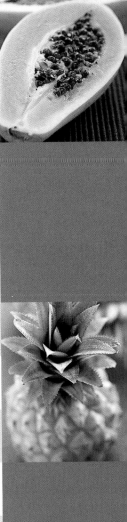

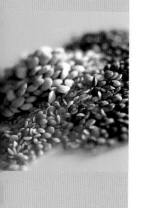

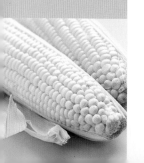

VEGETABLES	AVERAGE PORTION oz
Ackee, canned	2.8
Alfalfa sprouts	0.2
Artichoke, globe, heart	1.4
Artichoke, Jerusalem	2
Asparagus	4.4
Bamboo shoots, canned	1.8
Beans	
Aduki, dried, boiled	2
Baked, canned in tomato sauce	4.8
Baked, canned in tomato sauce, reduced sugar and salt	4.8
Balor, canned	4.8
Barbecue, canned in sauce	4.8
Blackeye, dried, boiled	2
Broad	4.2
Broad, canned	4.2
Broad, frozen	4.2
Butter, canned	4.2
Butter, dried, boiled	2
Chickpeas, canned	2.5
Chickpeas, split, dried, boiled	2.5
Chickpeas, whole, dried, boiled	2.5
Chili, canned	4.8
French	3.2
French, canned	3.2
French, frozen	3.2
Green	3.2
Green, canned	3.2
Green, frozen	3.2
Lilva, canned	2.8
Mung, dahl, dried, boiled	2
Navy, dried, boiled	2
Mung, whole, dried, boiled	2
Papri, canned	2

Unless otherwise stated, vegetables are described as they would normally be eaten.

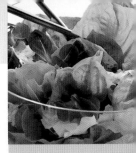

ENERGY cal	ENERGY J	FAT g	SATURATED FAT g	PROTEIN g	CARBOHYDRATE g	FIBER g
121	500	12	Trace	2	1	1.4
1	5	Trace	Trace	0	0	0.1
7	31	0	0	1	1	2
23	116	Trace	Trace	1	6	2
33	138	1	0.1	4	2	1.7
6	23	1	0.1	1	0	0.9
74	313	Trace	Trace	0	14	3.3
109	466	1	0.1	6	20	4.7
99	420	1	0.1	7	17	5.1
26	112	Trace	Trace	3	4	3.6
104	444	1	0.1	7	19	4.7
70	296	1	0.1	5	12	2.1
58	245	1	0.1	6	7	6.5
104	444	1	0.1	10	15	6.2
97	413	1	0.1	9	14	7.8
92	392	1	0.1	7	16	5.5
62	262	1	0.1	4	11	3.1
81	341	2	0.2	5	11	2.9
80	339	1	0.1	5	12	3
85	358	1	0.1	6	13	3
95	513	1	0.1	7	16	5.3
20	83	1	0.1	2	3	2.2
20	86	Trace	Trace	1	4	2.3
23	97	Trace	Trace	2	4	3.7
20	83	1	0.1	2	3	2.2
20	86	Trace	Trace	1	4	2.3
23	97	Trace	Trace	2	4	3.7
54	232	1	0.1	5	8	0.5
55	235	1	0.1	5	9	1.8
57	244	1	0.1	4	10	3.7
55	233	1	0.1	5	9	1.8
16	66	1	0.1	2	2	0.4

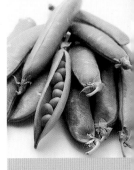

VEGETABLES
& SALADS 17

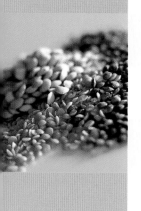

VEGETABLES	AVERAGE PORTION oz
Pigeon peas, dahl, dried	2
Pinto, dried, boiled	2
Pinto, refried	2
Red kidney, canned	2
Red kidney, dried, boiled	2
Runner	3.2
Soy, dried, boiled	2
Beansprouts, mung	2.8
Beansprouts, mung, canned	2.8
Beansprouts, mung, stir-fried	2.8
Beetroot	1.4
Beetroot, pickled	1.2
Belgian endive, raw	1
Bell peppers, green	5.6
Bell peppers, red	5.6
Bell peppers, yellow	5.6
Breadfruit, canned	1.4
Broccoli, green	3
Broccoli, purple sprouting	3
Brussels sprouts	3.2
Cabbage, Napa	1.4
Cabbage, red	3.2
Cabbage, red, raw	3.2
Cabbage, Savoy	3.4
Cabbage, white	3.4
Cabbage, white, raw	3.2
Carrots, canned	2
Carrots, old	2
Carrots, old, raw	2.8
Carrots, young	2
Carrots, young, raw	2
Cassava, baked	3.5
Cauliflower	3.2
Cauliflower, raw	3.2

Unless otherwise stated, vegetables are described as they would normally be eaten.

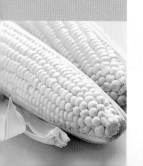

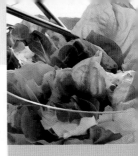

ENERGY cal	ENERGY J	FAT g	SATURATED FAT g	PROTEIN g	CARBOHYDRATE g	FIBER g
71	298	1	0.1	5	13	4
82	350	1	0.1	5	14	2.8
64	268	1	0.1	4	9	3.2
60	254	1	0.1	4	11	3.7
62	264	1	0.1	5	10	4
16	68	1	0.1	1	2	1.7
85	354	4	0.5	8	3	3.7
25	105	1	0.1	2	3	1.2
8	35	Trace	Trace	1	1	0.6
58	238	5	0.4	2	2	0.7
18	78	Trace	Trace	1	4	0.8
10	41	Trace	Trace	0	2	0.6
3	13	1	0.1	0	1	0.3
24	104	1	0.2	1	4	2.6
51	214	1	0.2	2	10	2.6
42	181	Trace	Trace	2	8	2.7
26	112	Trace	Trace	0	7	0.7
20	85	1	0.2	3	1	2
16	68	1	0.1	2	1	2
32	138	1	0.3	3	3	2.8
5	20	Trace	Trace	0	1	0.5
14	55	Trace	Trace	1	2	1.8
19	80	Trace	Trace	1	3	2.3
16	67	1	0.1	1	2	1.9
13	57	Trace	Trace	1	2	1.4
24	102	Trace	Trace	1	5	1.9
12	52	1	0.1	0	3	1.1
14	60	1	0.1	0	3	1.5
28	117	1	0.1	0	6	1.9
13	56	1	0.1	0	3	1.4
18	75	1	0.1	0	4	1.4
155	661	1	0.1	1	40	1.7
25	105	1	0.2	3	2	1.4
31	128	1	0.2	3	3	1.6

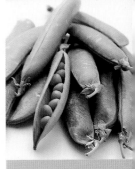

VEGETABLES & SALADS

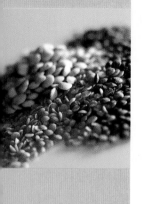

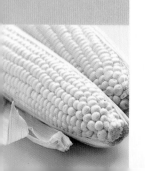

VEGETABLES	AVERAGE PORTION OZ
Celeriac (celery root)	1
Celeriac, raw	1
Celery	1
Chard, Swiss	3.2
Chili peppers, capsicum red	0.3
Chinese leaf	1.4
Corn, baby, canned	2
Corn kernels, canned, reheated	3
Corn, on the cob	7
Cucumber	0.8
Curly endive	1
Curly kale	3.4
Eggplant, fried	4.6
Fennel	1.4
Garlic, raw	0.1
Jackfruit, canned	2
Kohlrabi	2
Kohlrabi, cooked	3.2
Leeks	2.6
Lentils, canned in tomato sauce	2.8
Lentils, green or brown, whole, dried	2.8
Lentils, red, split, dried, boiled	2.8
Lettuce, Cos	2.8
Lettuce, Iceberg	2.8
Lettuce, Webbs Wonder	2.8
Mixed vegetables, frozen	3.2
Mushrooms	
Shiitake, steamed	1.4
Straw, canned	1.4
White, fried	1.5
White, raw	1.4
Okra	1
Onions	5.3
Onions, fried	1.4

Unless otherwise stated, vegetables are described as they would normally be eaten.

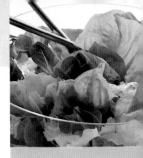

ENERGY cal	ENERGY J	FAT g	SATURATED FAT g	PROTEIN g	CARBOHYDRATE g	FIBER g
5	19	Trace	Trace	0	1	1
5	22	Trace	Trace	0	1	1.1
2	10	Trace	Trace	0	0	0.3
18	76	Trace	Trace	2	3	1.8
3	11	Trace	Trace	0	0	0.1
5	20	Trace	Trace	0	1	0.5
14	58	Trace	Trace	2	1	0.9
104	441	1	0.2	2	23	1.2
132	560	3	0.4	5	23	2.6
2	9	Trace	Trace	0	0	0.1
4	16	0	0	1	0	0.6
23	95	1	0.2	2	1	2.7
393	1620	41	5.3	2	4	3
5	20	Trace	Trace	0	1	1
3	12	0	0	0	0	0.1
62	264	Trace	Trace	0	16	0.9
14	57	Trace	Trace	1	2	1.3
16	69	Trace	Trace	1	3	1.7
16	65	1	0.1	1	2	1.3
44	189	Trace	Trace	4	7	1.4
84	357	1	0.1	7	14	3
80	339	Trace	Trace	6	14	1.5
13	52	1	0.1	1	1	1
10	42	Trace	Trace	1	2	0.5
10	44	Trace	Trace	1	2	0.6
38	162	Trace	Trace	3	6	2.9
22	93	Trace	0	1	5	0.8
6	25	Trace	Trace	1	0	1
69	284	7	0.9	1	0	0.7
5	22	Trace	0	1	0	0.4
8	36	1	0.1	1	1	1.1
54	225	Trace	Trace	2	12	2.1
66	274	4	0.6	1	6	1.2

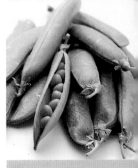

VEGETABLES & SALADS

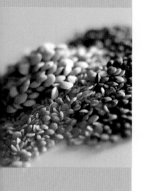

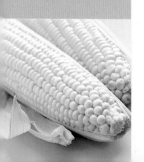

VEGETABLES	AVERAGE PORTION OZ
Parsnips	2.3
Parsnips, roasted without oil	3.2
Peas, canned	2.5
Peas, fresh	2.5
Peas, frozen	2.5
Peas, marrowfat, canned	2.8
Peas, petit pois, canned	2.5
Peas, petit pois, frozen	2.5
Peas, sugar-snap	3.2
Plantain	7
Plantain, ripe, fried	7
Potatoes and potato products	
Duchesse	4.2
Fries, crinkle cut, frozen, fried	5.8
Fries, frozen, baked	5.8
Fries, shoestring, frozen, fried	5.8
French fries	5.8
Fries, straight cut, frozen, fried	5.8
Microwave fries	5.8
Instant, made with low-fat milk	2
Instant, made with water	2
Instant, made with whole milk	2
New, canned	5.8
New, fried	5.8
New, in skins, boiled	6.2
Old, baked	6.3
Old, boiled	6.2
Old, mashed with butter	4.2
Old, mashed with polyunsaturated fat spread	4.2
Old, roasted	4.6
Steak fries, frozen, baked	5.8
Steak fries, frozen, fried	5.8

Unless otherwise stated, vegetables are described as they would normally be eaten.

ENERGY cal	ENERGY J	FAT g	SATURATED FAT g	PROTEIN g	CARBOHYDRATE g	FIBER g
43	181	1	0.1	1	8	3.1
102	427	6	Trace	1	12	4.2
56	237	1	0.1	4	9	3.6
55	230	1	0.2	5	7	3.2
48	204	1	0.1	4	7	3.6
80	329	1	0.1	6	14	3.3
32	132	1	0.1	4	3	3
34	144	1	0.1	4	4	3.2
30	125	1	0.1	3	4	1.2
224	954	1	0.2	2	57	2.4
534	2252	1	2	3	95	4.6
148	622	6	3.6	4	20	1.4
479	2001	28	5.1	6	55	3.6
267	1134	7	3	5	49	3.3
601	2515	35	6.6	7	68	4.5
312	1313	11	1.5	6	50	3.6
450	1889	22	4.1	7	59	4
365	1535	17	3	6	53	4.8
42	178	1	0.2	1	9	0.6
34	147	Trace	Trace	1	8	0.6
46	193	1	0.4	1	9	0.6
104	447	Trace	Trace	2	25	1.3
376	1582	16	2	7	55	2.8
116	492	1	0.2	2	27	2.6
245	1046	Trace	Trace	7	57	4.9
126	536	Trace	Trace	3	30	2.1
125	526	5	3.4	2	19	1.3
125	526	5	1.1	2	19	1.3
194	819	6	0.8	4	34	2.3
259	1096	7	2.8	5	46	3
386	1622	17	3.1	6	56	4

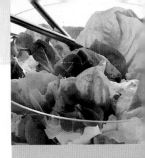

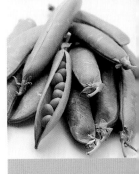

VEGETABLES & SALADS

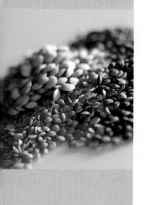

VEGETABLES	**AVERAGE PORTION oz**
Waffles, frozen	3.2
Wedges, baked	6.3
Pumpkin	2
Radicchio, raw	1
Radishes, red, raw	1.7
Rutabaga	2
Salad onions	0.3
Sauerkraut	1
Scallions	0.3
Snow peas, stir-fried	3.2
Spinach	3.2
Spinach, cooked	3.2
Split peas, dried, boiled	3.2
Spring greens, boiled	3.4
Squash, acorn, baked	2.3
Squash, butternut, baked	2.3
Squash, spaghetti, baked	2.3
Sweet potato	4.6
Sweet potato, baked	4.6
Tomatoes	3
Tomatoes, canned, not drained	7
Tomatoes, cherry	3.2
Tomatoes, fried	3
Tomatoes, grilled	3
Turnips	2
Water chestnuts, canned	1
Watercress	0.7
Yam	4.6
Yam, baked	4.6
Yam, steamed	4.6
Zucchini	3.2
Zucchini, fried	3.2

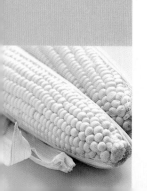

Unless otherwise stated, vegetables are described as they would normally be eaten.

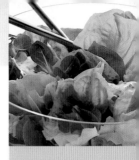

ENERGY cal	ENERGY J	FAT g	SATURATED FAT g	PROTEIN g	CARBOHYDRATE g	FIBER g
180	758	12	1	2	28	2
245	1046	Trace	Trace	7	57	4.9
8	34	1	0.1	0	1	0.7
4	17	Trace	Trace	0	1	0.5
6	24	0	0	0	1	0.4
7	28	Trace	Trace	0	1	0.4
2	10	0	0	0	0	0.2
3	11	Trace	Trace	0	0	0.7
2	10	0	0	0	0	0.2
64	268	4	0.4	3	3	2.2
23	93	1	0.1	3	1	1.9
17	71	1	0.1	2	1	1.9
113	484	1	0.2	7	20	2.4
19	78	1	0.1	2	2	2.5
36	152	Trace	Trace	1	8	2.1
21	89	Trace	Trace	1	5	0.9
15	62	Trace	0.1	0	3	1.4
109	465	1	0.1	1	27	3
150	634	1	0.3	2	36	4.3
14	62	1	0.1	1	3	0.9
32	138	Trace	Trace	2	6	1.4
16	68	1	0.1	1	3	0.9
77	320	7	0.9	1	4	1.1
42	179	1	0.3	2	8	2.5
7	31	1	Trace	0	1	1.1
9	37	Trace	Trace	0	3	2
4	19	1	0.1	1	0	0.3
173	738	1	0.1	2	43	1.8
199	846	1	0.1	3	49	2.2
148	634	1	0.1	2	37	1.7
17	73	1	0.1	2	2	1.1
57	239	4	0.5	2	2	1.1

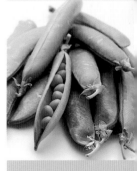

VEGETABLES
& SALADS **25**

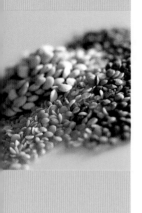

PREPARED SALADS

	AVERAGE PORTION oz
Arugula salad	1
Baby leaf salad	1.8
Bean salad	7
Beet salad	3.5
Caesar salad with chicken, no dressing	7.6
Caesar salad with shrimps, no dressing	8.2
Carrot and nut salad with French dressing	3.4
Coleslaw, with mayonnaise	3.5
Coleslaw, with reduced-calorie dressing	3.5
Coleslaw, with vinaigrette	3.5
Greek salad	3.4
Green salad	3.4
Herb salad	1.8
Pasta salad	3.4
Pasta salad, wholewheat	3.4
Potato salad, with mayonnaise	3
Potato salad, with reduced-calorie mayonnaise	3
Rice salad	3.2
Rice salad, brown	3.4
Taco salad	6.9
Tabbouleh	3.5
Tomato and onion salad	3.2
Vegetable salad, with shrimps, no dressing	8.2
Waldorf salad	3.2

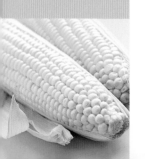

Unless otherwise stated, vegetables are described as they would normally be eaten.

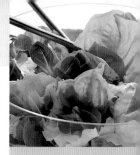

ENERGY cal	ENERGY J	FAT g	SATURATED FAT g	PROTEIN g	CARBOHYDRATE g	FIBER g
3	12	Trace	Trace	Trace	Trace	0.2
9	40	Trace	Trace	Trace	2	0.7
294	1236	19	2	8	26	6
100	417	7	0.7	2	8	1.7
105	438	2	0.6	17	4	1
106	444	2	0.7	15	7	1
207	858	17	1.6	2	13	2.3
258	939	26	3.9	1	4	1.4
67	280	5	0.5	1	6	1.4
87	364	4	0.5	1	12	1.7
124	513	12	3.1	3	2	0.8
11	48	0	Trace	1	2	1
9	40	Trace	Trace	Trace	Trace	0.7
121	473	7	1	2	13	1.5
124	493	7	1	3	13	2.6
203	757	18	2.6	1	10	0.8
82	349	3	0.3	1	13	0.7
149	628	7	1	3	21	0.6
159	668	7	1	3	23	1
279	1168	15	6.8	13	24	n/a
119	496	5	0.4	3	17	1
65	272	5	0.6	1	4	0.9
106	444	2	0.7	15	7	1
174	662	16	2.1	1	7	1.2

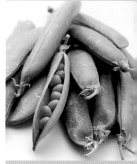

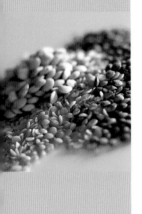

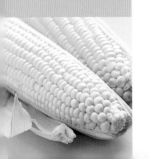

VEGETABLE DISHES, HOMEMADE	AVERAGE PORTION OZ
Bhaji pea, potato and cauliflower	2.5
Bhaji, potato and cauliflower, fried	2.5
Bhaji, potato and onion	2.5
Broccoli in cheese sauce, made with low-fat milk	6.7
Broccoli in cheese sauce, made with whole milk	6.7
Cannelloni, spinach	12
Cannelloni, vegetable	12
Casserole, vegetable	7.8
Cauliflower in cheese sauce, made with low-fat milk	7
Cauliflower in cheese sauce, made with whole milk	7
Cauliflower in white sauce, made with low-fat milk	7
Cauliflower in white sauce, made with whole milk	7
Chili, bean and lentil	10
Chili, vegetable	7.9
Curry, chickpea	7.4
Curry, potato and pea	10
Curry, vegetable	7
Dahl, mung bean, dried, boiled	2
Dahl, pigeon peas, dried, boiled	2
Falafel, fried	3.5
Lasagne, spinach	15
Lasagne, spinach, wholewheat	15
Lasagne, vegetable	15
Lasagne, vegetable, wholewheat	15
Moussaka, vegetable	11.6
Pakora, potato and cauliflower, fried	2.5
Peppers, stuffed with rice	6.2
Peppers, stuffed with vegetables,	

Unless otherwise stated, vegetables are described as they would normally be eaten.

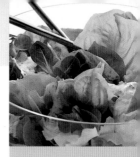

ENERGY cal	ENERGY J	FAT g	SATURATED FAT g	PROTEIN g	CARBOHYDRATE g	FIBER g
49	209	2	0.2	2	7	2
214	888	15	1.8	5	14	2.7
112	468	7	4.6	1	12	1.1
211	880	14	7.2	12	9	2.9
224	939	16	8.2	12	9	2.9
449	1880	26	7.8	15	43	2.7
493	2067	31	11.6	15	43	2.4
114	486	1	0.2	5	23	4.6
200	840	13	6	12	10	2.6
210	880	14	6.6	12	10	2.6
122	512	6	2.2	7	10	2.2
136	568	8	3.2	7	10	2.2
264	1111	8	0.9	15	38	10.4
125	532	1	0.2	7	24	5.7
227	956	9	0.8	13	30	6.9
267	1122	11	1.2	8	38	7
176	736	12	1.2	5	14	5
55	235	1	0.1	5	9	1.8
71	298	1	0.1	5	13	4
179	750	11	1.1	6	16	3.4
365	1541	13	5.5	15	53	4.6
391	1659	13	5.5	18	55	9.7
428	1810	18	9.2	17	52	4.2
445	1877	19	9.2	20	52	8.8
452	1888	31	9.2	15	30	4
214	888	15	1.8	5	14	2.7
149	630	4	0.7	3	27	2.3

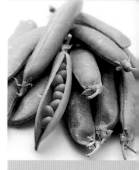

VEGETABLES & SALADS

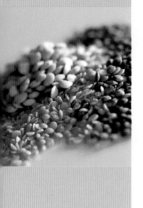

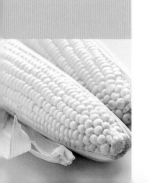

VEGETABLE DISHES, HOMEMADE	AVERAGE PORTION oz
cheese topping	6.2
Pilaf, mushroom	6.3
Pilaf, vegetable	6.3
Quiche, broccoli	5
Quiche, broccoli, wholewheat	5
Quiche, cauliflower and cheese	5
Quiche, cauliflower and cheese, wholewheat	5
Quiche, cheese and egg	5
Quiche, cheese and egg, wholewheat	5
Quiche, cheese and mushroom	5
Quiche, cheese and mushroom, wholewheat	5
Quiche, cheese, onion and potato	5
Quiche, cheese, onion and potato, wholewheat	5
Quiche, mushroom	5
Quiche, mushroom, wholewheat	5
Quiche, spinach	5
Quiche, spinach, wholewheat	5
Quiche, vegetable	5
Quiche, vegetable, wholewheat	5
Refried beans	3.2
Rice and blackeye beans	7
Rice and blackeye beans, brown rice	7
Risotto, vegetable	10
Risotto, vegetable, brown rice	10
Vegetable bake	9
Vine leaves, stuffed with rice	2.8

Unless otherwise stated, vegetables are described as they would normally be eaten.

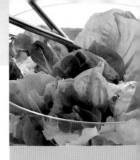

ENERGY cal	ENERGY J	FAT g	SATURATED FAT g	PROTEIN g	CARBOHYDRATE g	FIBER g
194	810	12	3.5	6	17	2.6
248	1048	8	4.5	4	43	0.7
248	1053	8	4.3	5	43	1
349	1455	21	8.3	12	30	1.7
337	1408	21	8.3	13	25	3.8
277	1156	18	7.1	7	24	1.5
269	1121	18	7.1	8	20	3.1
440	1834	31	14.4	18	24	0.8
431	1796	31	14.6	18	20	2.7
396	1655	26	10.8	15	26	1.3
388	1616	27	10.8	16	22	3.1
480	2005	33	16	18	28	1.4
472	1966	34	16.1	19	25	3.1
398	1659	27	12.2	14	26	1.3
388	1618	28	12.2	15	21	3.1
287	1203	18	5.6	14	18	2
281	1176	18	5.6	15	16	3.2
295	1238	18	6	7	28	2.1
286	1197	18	6	8	24	3.9
211	885	12	2.7	9	18	6.3
366	1556	7	3	12	68	2.8
350	1488	7	3	11	66	3.6
426	1798	19	2.9	12	56	6.4
415	1749	19	2.6	12	54	7
330	1383	18	7.8	11	32	2.9
210	875	14	2.1	2	19	1.0

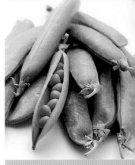

VEGETABLES & SALADS

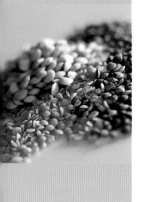

VEGETARIAN PRODUCTS & DISHES	AVERAGE PORTION oz
Beanburger, aduki, fried	3.2
Beanburger, butter bean, fried	3.2
Beanburger, red kidney bean, fried	3.2
Beanburger, soya, fried	3.2
Hormel vegetarian chili with beans, canned	8.7
Quorn™, myco-protein	3.2
Tempeh	2
Tofu, fried	2.8
Tofu, steamed	2.8
Tofu, steamed, fried	2.8
Tofu burger, baked	0.3
Vegeburger, fried	2
Vegeburger, grilled	2

Unless otherwise stated, vegetables are described as they would normally be eaten.

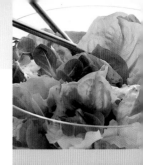

ENERGY cal	ENERGY J	FAT g	SATURATED FAT g	PROTEIN g	CARBOHYDRATE g	FIBER g
165	695	6	0.9	7	21	3.9
172	722	10	1.1	5	17	3.7
183	768	10	1.1	6	20	4.4
174	725	10	1.4	10	12	4.2
205	857	1	0.1	12	38	9.9
77	326	3	Trace	11	2	4.3
100	418	4	2	12	4	2.6
242	1011	20	2.3	17	3	1
58	243	3	0.4	6	1	1
209	869	14	2.3	19	2	1
11	45	0	0.1	1	1	0.2
137	571	10	1.7	9	4	2
110	460	6	1.7	9	4	2.4

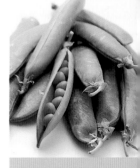

VEGETABLES
& SALADS

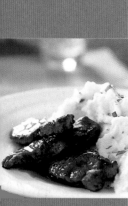

BEEF	AVERAGE PORTION OZ
Flank, choice, braised	3
Flank, choice, broiled	3
Flank, choice, lean and fat, braised	3
Flank, choice, lean and fat, broiled	3
Flank, pot roasted	5
Flank, untrimmed, pot roasted	5
Ground, extra lean, stewed	5
Ground, medium, extra lean, baked	3
Ground, medium, extra lean, broiled	3
Ground, medium, extra lean, pan-fried	3
Ground, medium, lean, baked	3
Ground, medium, lean, broiled	3
Ground, medium, lean, pan-fried	3
Ground, medium, regular, baked	3
Ground, medium, regular, broiled	3
Ground, medium, regular, pan-fried	3
Rib, large end, choice, braised	3
Rib, large end, choice, lean and fat, braised	3
Rib, large end, choice, lean and fat, $1/4$" fat, braised	3
Rib, large end, choice, $1/4$" fat, braised	3
Rib, large end, prime, lean and fat, $1/2$" fat, braised	3
Rib, large end, prime, lean and fat, $1/4$" fat, braised	3
Rib, large end, prime, $1/2$" fat, braised	3
Rib, large end, prime, $1/4$" fat, braised	3
Rib, large end, select, braised	3
Rib, large end, select, lean and fat, braised	3
Rib, large end, select, lean and fat, $1/4$" fat, braised	3
Rib, large end, select, $1/4$" fat, braised	3

Unless otherwise stated, all meat is lean and trimmed, and all chops and
cutlets are boned. Steaks are medium-sized. Unless stated otherwise, all
dishes are homemade.

ENERGY cal	ENERGY J	FAT g	SATURATED FAT g	PROTEIN g	CARBOHYDRATE g	FIBER g
201	843	11	4.7	24	0	0
176	736	9	3.7	23	0	0
224	935	14	5.9	23	0	0
192	804	11	4.5	22	0	0
354	1483	20	8	45	0	0
433	1800	31	12.7	38	0	0
248	1039	12	5.3	35	0	0
212	889	14	5.4	21	0	0
218	910	14	5.5	22	0	0
217	907	14	5.5	21	0	0
228	953	16	6.1	20	0	0
231	967	16	6.2	21	0	0
234	978	16	6.4	21	0	0
244	1021	18	7	20	0	0
246	1028	18	6.9	20	0	0
260	1088	19	7.5	20	0	0
215	900	13	5.1	23	0	0
316	1323	26	10.4	19	0	0
293	1227	26	10.8	13	0	0
204	853	12	5.1	21	0	0
326	1362	30	13	13	0	0
320	1340	29	12.3	13	0	0
250	1046	18	7.6	21	0	0
250	1046	18	7.6	21	0	0
187	782	10	3.9	23	0	0
281	1177	22	8.8	20	0	0
258	1081	22	9.1	14	0	0
175	733	9	3.8	21	0	0

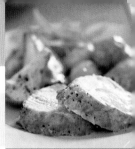

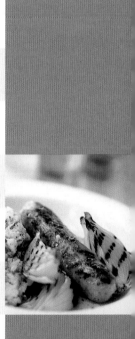

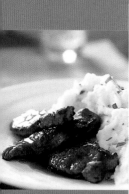

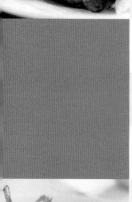

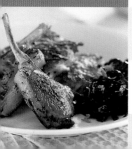

BEEF	**AVERAGE PORTION** oz
Rib, short, choice, braised	3
Rib, short, choice, lean and fat, braised	3
Rib, small end, choice, lean and fat, 1/4" fat, braised	3
Rib, small end, choice, 1/4" fat, braised	3
Rib, small end, prime, lean and fat, 1/2" fat, braised	3
Rib, small end, prime, lean and fat, 1/4" fat, braised	3
Rib, small end, prime, 1/2" fat, braised	3
Rib, small end, prime, 1/4" fat, braised	3
Rib roast, roasted	3.2
Rib roast, untrimmed, roasted	3.2
Short loin, porterhouse steak, choice, lean and fat, 1/4" fat, broiled	8
Short loin, porterhouse steak, choice, 1/4" fat, broiled	8
Short loin, porterhouse steak, select, lean and fat, 1/4" fat, broiled	8
Short loin, porterhouse steak, select, 1/4" fat, broiled	8
Short loin, t-bone steak, choice, lean and fat, 1/4" fat, broiled	8
Short loin, t-bone steak, choice, 1/4" fat, broiled	8
Short loin, t-bone steak, select, lean and fat, 1/4" fat, broiled	8

LAMB	
Leg, roasted medium	3.2
Leg, untrimmed, roasted medium	3.2
Leg, roasted well done	3.2
Leg, untrimmed, roasted well done	3.2

Unless otherwise stated, all meat is lean and trimmed, and all chops and
cutlets are boned. Steaks are medium-sized. Unless stated otherwise, all
dishes are homemade.

ENERGY cal	ENERGY J	FAT g	SATURATED FAT g	PROTEIN g	CARBOHYDRATE g	FIBER g
251	1049	15	6.6	26	0	0
400	1675	36	15.1	18	0	0
268	1120	23	9.4	14	0	0
137	573	7	2.7	17	0	0
297	1241	26	11.3	14	0	0
291	1216	26	10.6	14	0	0
221	925	13	5.6	24	0	0
221	925	13	5.6	24	0	0
212	889	10	4.6	30	0	0
270	1125	18	8.3	26	0	0
580	2428	45	18	40	0	0
360	1505	18	6.7	46	0	0
500	2090	33	13.5	47	0	0
335	1402	13	4.9	51	0	0
536	2241	39	15.7	42	0	0
461	1930	23	8.1	60	0	0
443	1854	28	11.5	44	0	0
183	768	8	3.4	27	0	0
216	904	13	5.3	25	0	0
187	786	8	3.3	28	0	0
218	909	12	5.1	27	0	0

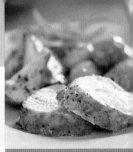

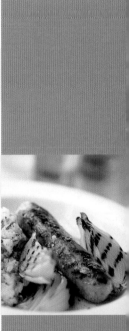

MEAT &
MEAT DISHES

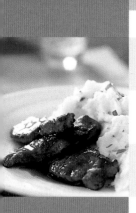

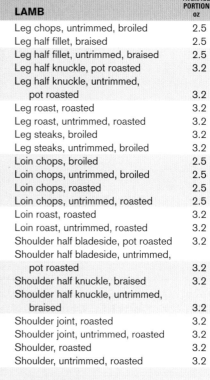

LAMB	AVERAGE PORTION oz
Leg chops, untrimmed, broiled	2.5
Leg half fillet, braised	2.5
Leg half fillet, untrimmed, braised	2.5
Leg half knuckle, pot roasted	3.2
Leg half knuckle, untrimmed, pot roasted	3.2
Leg roast, roasted	3.2
Leg roast, untrimmed, roasted	3.2
Leg steaks, broiled	3.2
Leg steaks, untrimmed, broiled	3.2
Loin chops, broiled	2.5
Loin chops, untrimmed, broiled	2.5
Loin chops, roasted	2.5
Loin chops, untrimmed, roasted	2.5
Loin roast, roasted	3.2
Loin roast, untrimmed, roasted	3.2
Shoulder half bladeside, pot roasted	3.2
Shoulder half bladeside, untrimmed, pot roasted	3.2
Shoulder half knuckle, braised	3.2
Shoulder half knuckle, untrimmed, braised	3.2
Shoulder joint, roasted	3.2
Shoulder joint, untrimmed, roasted	3.2
Shoulder, roasted	3.2
Shoulder, untrimmed, roasted	3.2

MEAT DISHES AND PRODUCTS

Beef bourguignon	9.2
Beef casserole, canned	9.5
Beef casserole, made with canned cook-in sauce	10.5
Beef pot pie, frozen	7

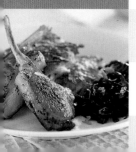

Unless otherwise stated, all meat is lean and trimmed, and all chops and
cutlets are boned. Steaks are medium-sized. Unless stated otherwise, all
dishes are homemade.

ENERGY cal	ENERGY J	FAT g	SATURATED FAT g	PROTEIN g	CARBOHYDRATE g	FIBER g
155	648	8	3.5	20	0	0
143	597	7	3.2	19	0	0
179	748	12	5.4	18	0	0
181	760	8	3.5	26	0	0
213	889	12	5.4	25	0	0
189	791	9	3.1	28	0	0
212	887	12	4.2	27	0	0
178	746	8	3.2	26	0	0
208	868	12	5	25	0	0
149	624	7	3.4	20	0	0
214	888	15	7.4	19	0	0
180	754	9	4.3	24	0	0
251	1043	19	9	20	0	0
188	788	10	4.4	25	0	0
273	1133	20	9.5	23	0	0
211	878	13	5.8	24	0	0
292	1212	23	10.8	21	0	0
191	797	11	4.9	23	0	0
272	1130	21	9.7	21	0	0
212	884	12	5.6	26	0	0
254	1056	18	8.4	23	0	0
196	819	11	5	24	0	0
268	1114	20	9.4	22	0	0
328	1368	17	5.5	36	7	1
211	886	7	3.8	19	19	2.7
408	1707	20	8.1	45	14	2.7
449	1881	24	8.5	13	44	2.2

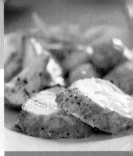

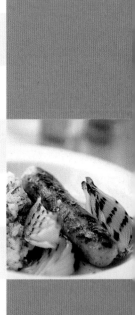

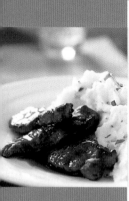

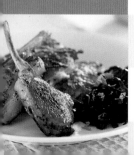

MEAT DISHES AND PRODUCTS	AVERAGE PORTION OZ
Beef sausages, fried	1.4
Beef sausages, broiled	1.4
Beef stew	9.8
Beef stew, made with lean beef	9.2
Beef stew and dumplings	9.2
Bologna, beef	1.6
Bologna, beef and pork	1.6
Bologna, pork	1.6
Bratwurst	2.6
Chili con carne	7.8
Chili con carne, canned	7.9
Chili con carne, store bought	7.8
Chili with beans, canned	9
Chorizo	1
Corned beef	1.8
Corned beef, brisket, cooked	3
Corned beef, canned	1.9
Corned beef hash	10.5
Corned beef loaf, jellied	1.9
El Rio chili, no beans, canned	9.2
Enchilada, with cheese	5.4
Enchilada, with cheese and beef	6.7
Hamburgers, broiled	3.5
Hamburgers, fried	3.5
Hamburgers, broiled	3.5
Hamburgers, low-fat, fried	3.5
Hamburgers, low-fat, broiled	3.5
Hamburgers in gravy, canned	3.5
Hormel chili with beans, canned	8.7
Hormel chili, no beans, canned	8.3
Hormel, Wrangler beef franks	3.9
Lebanon bologna, beef	46
Liver sausage/wurst, pork	1.2
Meatloaf	3.5

Unless otherwise stated, all meat is lean and trimmed, and all chops and
cutlets are boned. Steaks are medium-sized. Unless stated otherwise, all
dishes are homemade.

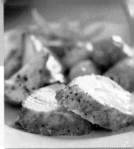

ENERGY cal	ENERGY J	FAT g	SATURATED FAT g	PROTEIN g	CARBOHYDRATE g	FIBER g
112	464	8	3	5	5	0.3
111	463	8	3.2	5	5	0.3
316	1328	14	4.2	34	14	2
263	1102	9	2.3	32	13	1.8
499	2090	27	12.5	26	41	2.6
144	600	13	5.6	6	0	0
145	608	13	4.9	5	1	0
114	475	9	3.2	7	0	0
195	811	16	6	12	2	Trace
286	1199	17	6.6	20	10	2.4
255	1068	8	2.1	20	24	8.2
211	889	9	4.2	17	16	3.1
287	1201	14	6	15	30	11.3
87	362	7	2.9	5	1	Trace
103	430	5	2.8	13	1	0
213	892	16	5.4	15	0	0
140	586	8	3.5	15	0	0
423	1776	18	9.9	31	37	3
87	365	3	1.5	13	0	0
305	1279	20	7.5	15	16	3.7
319	1337	19	10.6	10	29	n/a
323	1350	18	9	12	30	n/a
326	1355	24	10.9	27	0	0
303	1261	23	8.7	24	1	0.2
287	1194	20	8.8	25	1	0.2
193	807	11	5	24	0	0
178	745	10	4.4	23	1	0
171	713	12	4.8	12	5	Trace
240	1003	4	1.8	17	34	8.4
194	809	7	2.2	17	18	3.1
325	1360	29	11.9	14	2	0
98	408	6	2.7	9	1	0
117	491	10	3.8	5	1	0
214	894	11	4.1	17	13	0.5

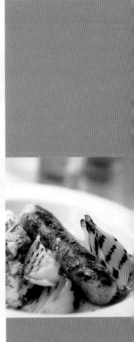

MEAT &
MEAT DISHES

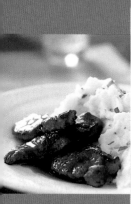

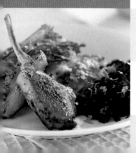

MEAT DISHES AND PRODUCTS	AVERAGE PORTION OZ
Mortadella	0.8
Moussaka	11.6
Moussaka, store bought	11.6
Nalley chili con carne, canned	9.1
Nestlé, Chef-Mate chili with beans, canned	8.9
Nestlé, Chef-Mate chili without beans, canned	8.8
Nestlé, Chef-Mate spicy chili with beans, canned	8.9
Old El Paso chili with beans, canned	7.9
Oscar Mayer wieners	1.6
Oscar Mayer wieners (bun length)	2
Oscar Mayer wieners, fat free	1.7
Oscar Mayer wieners, light	2
Pastrami	1.8
Pork and beef meatballs in tomato sauce	5.6
Pork and beef sausages, broiled	1.4
Pork casserole, made with canned cook-in sauce	9.2
Pork, cured, ham, patties, broiled	2
Pork sausages, fried	1.4
Pork sausages, broiled	1.4
Pork sausages, frozen, fried	1.4
Pork sausages, frozen, broiled	1.4
Pork sausages, reduced-fat, fried	1.4
Pork sausages, reduced-fat, broiled	1.4
Premium sausages, fried	1.4
Premium sausages, broiled	1.4
Stagg classic chili with beans, canned	8.7
Stagg country chili with beans, canned	8.7
Stagg Dynamite chili with beans, canned	8.7

Unless otherwise stated, all meat is lean and trimmed, and all chops and
cutlets are boned. Steaks are medium-sized. Unless stated otherwise, all
dishes are homemade.

ENERGY cal	ENERGY J	FAT g	SATURATED FAT g	PROTEIN g	CARBOHYDRATE g	FIBER g
79	328	7	2.8	3	0	Trace
403	1680	26	11.9	28	15	3.3
462	1934	27	9.6	27	28	2.6
281	1176	8	2.8	40	12	12.9
412	1725	25	10.9	18	29	11.1
430	1800	32	14.4	19	18	3
423	1768	25	10.7	17	33	4.3
249	1040	10	2.1	18	22	9.8
143	599	13	5.6	5	1	0
184	768	17	7.1	6	2	0
39	163	0	0.1	7	3	0
110	461	8	3.6	6	2	0
62	259	2	0.9	10	1	0
202	840	12	4.4	16	8	1.2
108	448	8	3	5	4	0.5
398	1664	20	6.8	44	10	0
205	859	19	6.7	8	1	0
123	512	10	3.4	6	4	0.3
118	488	9	3.2	6	4	0.3
126	525	10	3.5	6	4	0.3
116	482	8	3	6	4	0.3
84	352	5	1.7	6	4	0.6
92	384	6	2	6	4	0.6
110	457	8	3.1	6	3	0.3
117	486	9	3.3	7	3	0.3
324	1354	16	6.7	17	29	7.4
319	1334	16	6.8	15	29	5.9
333	1396	15	5.7	18	31	8.2

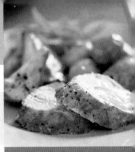

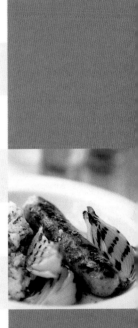

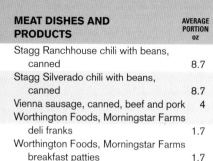

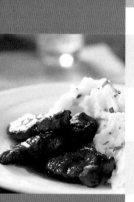

MEAT DISHES AND PRODUCTS	AVERAGE PORTION OZ
Stagg Ranchhouse chili with beans, canned	8.7
Stagg Silverado chili with beans, canned	8.7
Vienna sausage, canned, beef and pork	4
Worthington Foods, Morningstar Farms deli franks	1.7
Worthington Foods, Morningstar Farms breakfast patties	1.7

VARIETY MEATS

Heart, beef, stewed	7
Heart, lamb, roasted	7
Heart, lamb, stewed	7
Heart, pork, stewed	3.5
Kidney, beef, stewed	4
Kidney, lamb, fried	1.3
Kidney, pork, fried	5
Kidney, pork, stewed	5
Liver, beef, stewed	2.5
Liver, calf, fried	3.5
Liver, chicken, fried	2.5
Liver, lamb, fried	2.5
Liver, pork, stewed	2.5

PORK, BACON AND HAM
Bacon

Hormel Canadian style bacon	2
Pork, cured, bacon, broiled, pan-fried or roasted	0.7
Pork, cured, Canadian-style bacon, grilled	1.7

Unless otherwise stated, all meat is lean and trimmed, and all chops and cutlets are boned. Steaks are medium-sized. Unless stated otherwise, all dishes are homemade.

ENERGY cal	ENERGY J	FAT g	SATURATED FAT g	PROTEIN g	CARBO-HYDRATE g	FIBER g
284	1188	9	2.6	19	32	8.6
227	951	3	1	18	33	8.2
315	1319	28	10.5	12	2	0
112	467	6	0.9	10	4	2.7
79	332	3	0.5	10	4	2
314	1322	10	5	56	0	0
452	1888	28	6.2	51	0	0
312	1308	15	6	24	20	0
162	678	7	1.3	25	0	0
155	648	5	1.6	27	0	0
66	274	4	0.4	8	0	0
283	1187	13	2.1	41	0	0
214	897	9	2.8	34	0	0
139	582	7	2.5	17	2	0
176	734	10	2.7	22	Trace	0
118	494	6	3.5	15	Trace	0
237	989	13	4.9	30	Trace	0
132	555	6	1.8	18	2	0
68	286	3	1	9	1	0
109	458	9	3.3	6	0	0
87	364	4	1.3	11	1	0

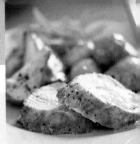
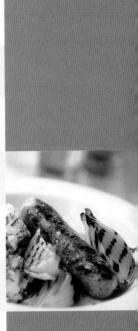

MEAT &
MEAT DISHES

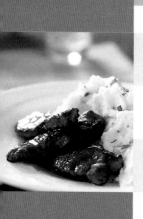

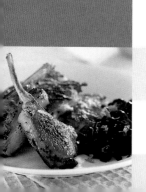

PORK, BACON AND HAM	AVERAGE PORTION OZ
Blade chops, bone-in, braised	3
Blade chops, bone-in, broiled	3
Blade chops, bone-in, lean and fat, braised	3
Blade chops, bone-in, lean and fat, broiled	3
Blade chops, bone-in, lean and fat, pan-fried	3
Blade chops, bone-in, pan-fried	3
Blade roast, bone-in, lean and fat, roasted	3
Blade roast, bone-in, roasted	3
Boston blade roast, lean and fat, roasted	3
Boston blade roast, roasted	3
Boston blade steak, braised	3
Boston blade steak, broiled	3
Boston blade steak, lean and fat, braised	3
Boston blade steak, lean and fat, broiled	3
Center loin chops, bone-in, braised	3
Center loin chops, bone-in, broiled	3
Center loin chops, bone-in, lean and fat, braised	3
Center loin chops, bone-in, lean and fat, broiled	3
Center loin chops, bone-in, lean and fat, pan-fried	3
Center loin chops, bone-in, pan-fried	3
Center loin rib roast, bone-in, lean and fat, roasted	3
Center loin rib roast, bone-in, roasted	3
Center loin rib roast, lean and fat, roasted	3
Center loin rib roast, roasted	3
Center loin roast, bone-in, lean and fat, roasted	3
Center loin roast, bone-in, roasted	3

Unless otherwise stated, all meat is lean and trimmed, and all chops and cutlets are boned. Steaks are medium-sized. Unless stated otherwise, all dishes are homemade.

ENERGY cal	ENERGY J	FAT g	SATURATED FAT g	PROTEIN g	CARBOHYDRATE g	FIBER g
191	800	11	4	21	0	0
199	832	12	4.3	22	0	0
275	1148	22	8.1	19	0	0
272	1138	21	7.9	19	0	0
291	1216	24	8.6	18	0	0
205	857	13	4.4	21	0	0
275	1148	21	7.8	20	0	0
210	878	13	4.5	23	0	0
229	956	16	5.9	20	0	0
197	825	12	4.4	21	0	0
232	971	13	4.7	26	0	0
193	808	11	3.8	23	0	0
271	1135	18	6.7	24	0	0
220	921	14	5.1	22	0	0
172	718	7	2.6	25	0	0
172	718	7	2.5	26	0	0
210	878	12	4.5	24	0	0
204	853	11	4.1	24	0	0
235	985	14	5.1	25	0	0
197	825	9	3.1	27	0	0
217	907	13	5	23	0	0
190	793	9	3.7	24	0	0
214	896	13	4.5	23	0	0
182	761	9	3	24	0	0
199	832	11	4.3	22	0	0
169	708	8	2.8	23	0	0

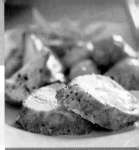

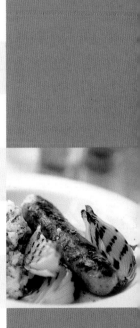

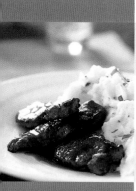

PORK, BACON AND HAM	AVERAGE PORTION OZ
Center rib chops, bone-in, braised	3
Center rib chops, bone-in, broiled	3
Center rib chops, bone-in, lean and fat, braised	3
Center rib chops, bone-in, lean and fat, broiled	3
Center rib chops, bone-in, lean and fat, pan-fried	3
Center rib chops, bone-in, pan-fried	3
Center rib chops, braised	3
Center rib chops, braised	3
Center rib chops, braised	3
Center rib chops, broiled	3
Center rib chops, broiled	3
Center rib chops, lean and fat, braised	3
Center rib chops, lean and fat, broiled	3
Center rib chops, lean and fat, broiled	3
Center rib chops, lean and fat, pan-fried	3
Center rib chops, pan-fried	3
Ham	
Ham, canned	3.2
Ham, Parma	1.7
Ham, premium	2
Pork shoulder, cured	3.5
Loin, whole, braised	3
Loin, whole, broiled	3
Loin, whole, lean and fat, braised	3
Loin, whole, lean and fat, broiled	3
Loin, whole, lean and fat, roasted	3
Loin, whole, roasted	3
Ribs, country-style, braised	3
Ribs, country-style, lean and fat, braised	3
Ribs, country-style, lean and fat, roasted	3
Ribs, country-style, roasted	3

Unless otherwise stated, all meat is lean and trimmed, and all chops and cutlets are boned. Steaks are medium-sized. Unless stated otherwise, all dishes are homemade.

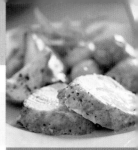

ENERGY cal	ENERGY J	FAT g	SATURATED FAT g	PROTEIN g	CARBOHYDRATE g	FIBER g
175	733	8	3.1	24	0	0
186	779	8	2.9	26	0	0
212	889	13	5	23	0	0
224	935	13	4.8	24	0	0
225	943	14	5.4	22	0	0
185	775	9	3.4	24	0	0
179	751	9	3.4	24	0	0
179	751	9	3.4	24	0	0
179	751	9	3.4	24	0	0
184	768	9	3	25	0	0
184	768	9	3	25	0	0
217	907	13	5.2	22	0	0
221	925	13	4.9	23	0	0
221	925	13	4.9	23	0	0
190	796	10	3.7	24	0	0
190	796	10	3.7	24	0	0
96	404	4	1.4	15	0	0
105	438	6	2	13	Trace	Trace
74	310	3	1	12	0	0
103	435	4	1.2	17	1	0
173	726	8	2.9	24	0	0
178	747	8	3.1	24	0	0
203	850	12	4.3	23	0	0
206	861	12	4.4	23	0	0
211	882	12	4.6	23	0	0
178	743	8	3	24	0	0
199	832	12	4.2	22	0	0
252	1052	18	6.8	20	0	0
279	1166	22	7.8	20	0	0
210	878	13	4.5	23	0	0

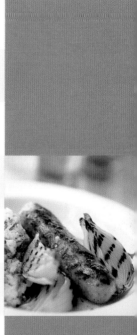

MEAT &
MEAT DISHES

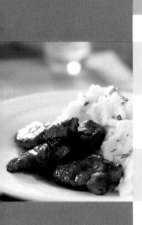

PORK, BACON AND HAM

	AVERAGE PORTION oz
Shoulder, arm picnic, braised	3
Shoulder, arm picnic, lean and fat, braised	3
Shoulder, arm picnic, lean and fat, roasted	3
Shoulder, arm picnic, roasted	3
Shoulder, whole, lean and fat, roasted	3
Shoulder, whole, roasted	3
Spare ribs, lean and fat, braised	3
Tenderloin, broiled	3
Tenderloin, lean and fat, broiled	3
Tenderloin, lean and fat, roasted	3
Tenderloin, roasted	3
Top loin chops, braised	3
Top loin chops, broiled	3
Top loin chops, lean and fat, braised	3
Top loin chops, lean and fat, broiled	3
Top loin chops, lean and fat, pan-fried	3
Top loin chops, pan-fried	3
Top loin roast, lean and fat, roasted	3
Top loin roast, roasted	3

VEAL

Ground, broiled	3
Rib, braised	3
Rib, lean and fat, braised	3
Rib, lean and fat, roasted	3
Rib, roasted	3
Shank (fore and hind), braised	3
Shank (fore and hind), lean and fat, braised	3
Sirloin, braised	3
Sirloin, lean and fat, braised	3
Sirloin, lean and fat, roasted	3
Sirloin, roasted	3

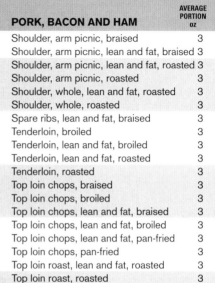

Unless otherwise stated, all meat is lean and trimmed, and all chops and cutlets are boned. Steaks are medium-sized. Unless stated otherwise, all dishes are homemade.

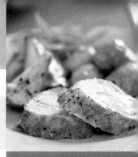

ENERGY cal	ENERGY J	FAT g	SATURATED FAT g	PROTEIN g	CARBOHYDRATE g	FIBER g
211	882	10	3.5	27	0	0
280	1170	20	7.2	24	0	0
269	1127	20	7.5	20	0	0
194	811	11	3.7	23	0	0
248	1039	18	6.7	20	0	0
196	818	12	4.1	22	0	0
337	1412	26	9.5	25	0	0
159	665	5	1.9	26	0	0
171	715	7	2.5	25	0	0
147	615	5	1.8	24	0	0
139	583	4	1.4	24	0	0
172	718	7	2.7	25	0	0
173	722	7	2.3	26	0	0
198	829	11	4	24	0	0
195	814	10	3.4	25	0	0
218	914	13	4.5	25	0	0
191	800	9	3.1	26	0	0
192	804	10	3.5	24	0	0
165	690	6	2.2	26	0	0
146	612	6	2.6	21	0	0
185	775	7	2.2	29	0	0
213	892	11	4.2	28	0	0
194	811	12	4.6	20	0	0
150	630	6	1.8	22	0	0
150	630	4	1	27	0	0
162	679	5	1.8	27	0	0
173	726	6	1.5	29	0	0
214	896	11	4.4	27	0	0
172	718	9	3.8	21	0	0
143	598	5	2	22	0	0

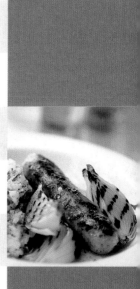

MEAT &

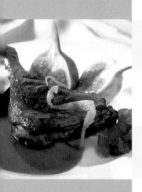

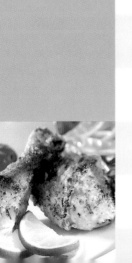

CHICKEN	AVERAGE PORTION oz
Breast, broiled	4.6
Breast, broiled and skinned	4.6
Breast, casseroled	4.6
Breast, flour-coated, fried	3.5
Breast, fried in batter	5
Breast, skinned, broiled	4.6
Breast, skinned, casseroled	4.6
Breast, skinned, fried	3
Breast strips, stir-fried	3.2
Corn-fed chicken, dark meat, roasted	3.2
Corn-fed chicken, light meat, roasted	3.2
Dark meat, flour-coated, fried	3.9
Dark meat, fried in batter	5.8
Dark meat, roasted	3.5
Dark meat, skinned, fried	3.3
Drumsticks, casseroled	1.7
Drumsticks, flour-coated, fried	1.8
Drumsticks, fried in batter	2.6
Drumsticks, roasted	1.7
Drumsticks, skinned, casseroled	1.7
Drumsticks, skinned, fried	1.5
Drumsticks, skinned, roasted	1.7
Leg, flour-coated, fried	4
Leg, fried in batter	5.5
Leg quarter, casseroled	5.2
Leg quarter, roasted	5.2
Leg quarter, skinned, casseroled	5.2
Leg, skinned, fried	3.3
Light meat, flour-coated, fried	4.6
Light meat, fried in batter	4
Light meat, roasted	3.5
Light meat, skinned, fried	3.5
Thighs, casseroled	1.6
Thighs, flour-coated, fried	2.2

Unless otherwise stated, chicken and turkey are neither skinned nor
boned, game is skinned and trimmed and dishes are homemade.

ENERGY cal	ENERGY J	FAT g	SATURATED FAT g	PROTEIN g	CARBOHYDRATE g	FIBER g
225	946	8	1.2	38	0	0
191	807	4	1.2	39	0	0
239	1004	11	3.1	35	0	0
218	910	9	2.4	31	2	0.1
364	1523	18	4.9	35	13	0.4
192	814	4	0.8	42	0	0
148	628	7	2	37	0	0
161	673	4	1.1	29	0	0
145	609	4	0.8	27	0	0
167	695	9	2.5	22	0	0
127	536	4	1.1	23	0	0
314	1311	19	5	30	4	0
498	2082	31	8.3	36	16	0
196	819	11	2.9	24	0	0
217	910	11	2.8	26	2	0
102	425	7	1.8	10	0	0
120	502	7	1.8	13	1	0
193	807	11	3	16	6	0.2
87	364	4	1.2	12	0	0
87	363	5	1.2	11	0	0
82	343	3	0.9	12	0	0
71	301	2	0.7	13	0	0
284	1191	16	4.4	30	3	0.1
431	1804	26	6.8	34	14	0.5
317	1320	20	5.5	33	0	0
345	1432	25	6.7	31	0	0
257	1075	12	3.4	37	0	0
196	818	9	2.3	27	1	0
320	1338	16	4.3	40	2	0.1
313	1310	17	4.7	27	11	0
153	645	4	1	30	0	0
192	803	6	1.5	33	0	0
105	436	7	2	10	0	0
162	680	9	2.5	17	2	0.1

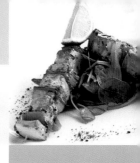

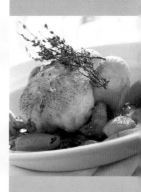

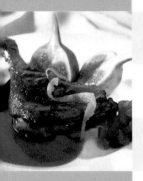
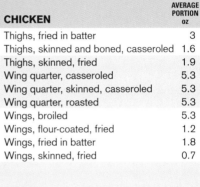

CHICKEN

	AVERAGE PORTION oz
Thighs, fried in batter	3
Thighs, skinned and boned, casseroled	1.6
Thighs, skinned, fried	1.9
Wing quarter, casseroled	5.3
Wing quarter, skinned, casseroled	5.3
Wing quarter, roasted	5.3
Wings, broiled	5.3
Wings, flour-coated, fried	1.2
Wings, fried in batter	1.8
Wings, skinned, fried	0.7

CHICKEN PRODUCTS AND DISHES

Chicken and mushroom pie, single crust	3.5
Chicken curry	12.3
Chicken curry, with bone	12.3
Chicken curry, without bone	10.6
Chicken fingers, baked	3.2
Chicken goujons, baked	3.2
Chicken in crumbs, stuffed with cheese and vegetables, baked	3.5
Chicken in sauce with vegetables	10.2
Chicken in white sauce, canned	3.5
Chicken in white sauce, made with low-fat milk	7
Chicken in white sauce, made with whole milk	7
Chicken Kiev, frozen, baked	6
Chicken pie, individual, baked	4.6
Chicken risotto	12.3
Curry chicken salad	7
Frankfurter, chicken	1.6
Lemon chicken	3.5
Tandoori chicken	3.5

Unless otherwise stated, chicken and turkey are neither skinned nor boned, game is skinned and trimmed and dishes are homemade.

ENERGY cal	ENERGY J	FAT g	SATURATED FAT g	PROTEIN g	CARBOHYDRATE g	FIBER g
238	997	14	3.8	19	8	0.3
81	340	4	1.1	12	0	0
113	474	5	1.4	15	1	0
315	1316	19	5.3	37	0	0
246	1035	9	2.6	40	0	0
339	1415	21	5.9	37	0	0
274	1146	17	4.6	27	Trace	0
103	430	7	1.9	8	1	0
159	664	11	2.9	10	5	0.1
42	177	2	0.5	6	0	0
200	836	10	4.5	13	14	0.6
522	2174	31	14	42	19	4.5
539	2237	44	6	27	8	2.4
615	2550	51	6.6	31	9	2.7
185	774	9	2.7	11	17	Trace
249	1045	13	3.6	17	18	0.6
230	963	14	4.1	16	11	0.9
336	1412	15	7	39	13	0.9
141	590	8	2.3	14	3	Trace
310	1298	16	5	34	10	0.2
328	1376	18	6.2	34	10	0.2
456	1902	29	12.1	32	19	1
374	1563	21	9.1	12	32	1
546	2310	10	4.5	31	84	Trace
728	3012	63	10.4	33	6	Trace
116	484	9	2.5	6	3	0
155	652	6	0.8	16	9	Trace
214	897	11	3.3	27	2	Trace

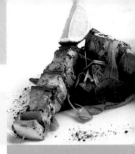

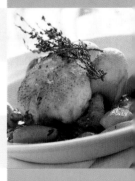

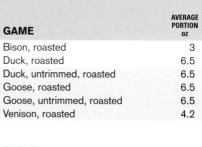

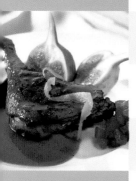

GAME	AVERAGE PORTION oz
Bison, roasted	3
Duck, roasted	6.5
Duck, untrimmed, roasted	6.5
Goose, roasted	6.5
Goose, untrimmed, roasted	6.5
Venison, roasted	4.2

TURKEY	
Breast, broiled and skinned	3.2
Dark meat, roasted	3.2
Drumsticks, roasted	3.2
Drumsticks, roasted and skinned	3.2
Light meat, roasted	3.2
Light meat, from self-basting bird, roasted	3.2
Strips, stir-fried	3.2
Thighs, skinned and boned, casseroled	3.2

TURKEY PRODUCTS	
Frankfurter, turkey	1.6
Louis Rich, honey roasted, fat-free bird	1.8
Louis Rich, turkey bacon	1
Louis Rich, turkey bologna	1
Louis Rich, turkey salami	1
Louis Rich, turkey smoked sausage	1.8
Oscar Mayer, Smokies sausage little	1.9
Oscar Mayer, wieners	1.9
Oscar Mayer, wieners	1.6
Pastrami, turkey	1
Pot pie, frozen	14
Salami, turkey	1
Turkey patties, breaded, battered, fried	2.3

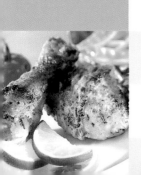

Unless otherwise stated, chicken and turkey are neither skinned nor boned, game is skinned and trimmed and dishes are homemade.

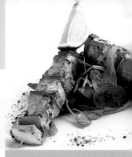

ENERGY cal	ENERGY J	FAT g	SATURATED FAT g	PROTEIN g	CARBOHYDRATE g	FIBER g
122	508	2	0.8	24	0	0
361	1508	19	6.1	47	0	0
783	3238	92	21.1	37	0	0
590	2455	41	13.7	54	0	0
557	2316	39	12.2	51	0	0
198	838	3	1	43	0	0
140	592	2	0.5	32	0	0
159	671	6	1.8	26	0	0
167	702	8	2.3	25	0	0
146	615	5	1.5	25	0	0
138	583	2	0.6	30	0	0
147	619	4	1.1	29	0	0
148	623	4	1.1	28	0	0
163	684	7	2.3	25	0	0
102	426	8	2.7	6	1	0
57	239	0	0.1	11	3	0
68	286	5	1.5	4	1	0
52	216	4	1.1	3	1	0
41	172	3	0.8	4	0	0
90	375	5	1.5	8	2	0
172	718	15	5.4	7	1	0
111	463	8	3	7	2	0
145	606	13	4.3	5	1	0
82	342	4	1	11	1	0
699	2922	35	11.4	26	70	4.4
114	476	8	2.3	9	0	0
181	758	12	3	9	10	0.3

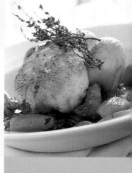

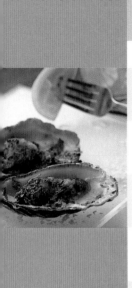

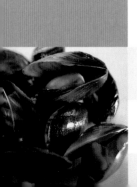

FISH	AVERAGE PORTION oz
Anchovies, canned in oil	0.4
Cod, baked	4.2
Cod, coated in batter, frozen, baked	6.3
Cod, coated in crumbs, frozen, fried	3.5
Cod, dried, salted, boiled	3.2
Cod, frozen, grilled	4.2
Cod, in batter, fried	6.3
Cod, in parsley sauce, frozen, boiled	6
Cod, poached	4.2
Cod, smoked, poached	4.2
Cod, steamed	4.2
Conger eel, grilled	4
Dogfish, in batter, fried	4.4
Haddock, grilled	4.2
Haddock, in batter, fried	4.2
Haddock, in crumbs, fried	4.2
Haddock, in crumbs, frozen, fried	4.2
Haddock, in flour, fried	4.2
Haddock, poached	4.2
Haddock, smoked, poached	5.3
Haddock, smoked, steamed	5.3
Haddock, steamed	4.2
Hake, grilled	3.5
Halibut, grilled	4.2
Halibut, poached	3.9
Halibut, steamed	3.9
Herring, grilled	4.2
Herring, pickled	3.2
Hoki, grilled	6.7
Kipper, baked	6.6
Kipper, grilled	4.6
Lemon sole, grilled	3.8
Lemon sole, in crumbs, fried	3.8
Lemon sole, steamed	3.8

Unless otherwise stated, values for bottled and canned seafood are for drained weights.

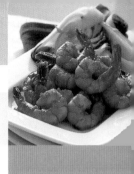

ENERGY cal	ENERGY J	FAT g	SATURATED FAT g	PROTEIN g	CARBOHYDRATE g	FIBER g
28	117	2	0.4	3	0	0
115	490	1	0.4	26	Trace	0
380	1589	21	6.5	23	26	1.1
235	983	14	1.5	12	15	0.4
124	527	1	0.2	29	0	0
114	482	2	0.5	25	Trace	0
445	1856	28	7.4	29	21	0.9
143	598	5	3	20	5	0.2
113	475	1	0.4	25	Trace	0
121	511	2	0.7	26	Trace	0
100	420	1	0.2	22	0	0
158	660	6	Trace	25	0	0
369	1531	27	6.6	18	13	0.5
125	530	1	0.2	29	0	0
278	1163	17	4.4	21	12	0.5
209	875	10	0.8	26	4	0.2
235	986	12	1	18	15	0.7
166	698	5	0.5	25	5	0.2
136	572	5	3.1	21	1	0
201	843	9	5.6	28	2	0
152	644	1	0.3	35	0	0
107	454	1	0.1	25	0	0
113	478	3	0.4	22	0	0
175	744	3	0.6	37	0	0
169	713	6	3	27	1	0
144	608	4	0.6	26	0	0
215	900	13	3.3	24	0	0
188	789	10	3.3	15	9	0
230	969	5	1	46	0	0
267	1112	15	2.3	33	0	0
332	1378	25	4	26	0	0
106	445	2	0.2	22	0	0
235	985	14	1.4	18	10	0.4
99	419	1	0.1	22	0	0

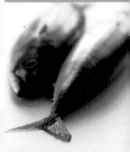

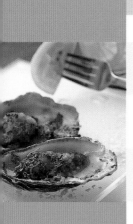

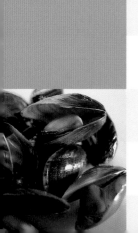

FISH	AVERAGE PORTION OZ
Lemon sole, strips, baked	6
Lemon sole, strips, fried	6
Lobster, boiled, dressed with shell	8.8
Mackerel, canned in brine	7
Mackerel, canned in tomato sauce	4.4
Mackerel, fried	5.7
Mackerel, grilled	5.2
Mackerel, smoked	5.3
Monkfish, grilled	2.5
Mullet, Grey, grilled	3.5
Mullet, Red, grilled	3.5
Plaice, frozen, grilled	5.8
Plaice, frozen, steamed	4.6
Plaice, goujons, baked	4.6
Plaice, goujons, fried	5.3
Plaice, grilled	4.6
Plaice, in batter, fried	7
Plaice, in crumbs, fried	5.3
Plaice, in crumbs, frozen, fried	5.3
Plaice, steamed	4.6
Red snapper, fried	3.6
Rock salmon, in batter, fried	4.4
Salmon, grilled	2.9
Salmon, pink, canned in brine, skinned and boned	3.5
Salmon, raw	3.5
Salmon, red, canned in brine, skinned and boned	3.5
Salmon, smoked	2
Salmon, steamed	2.7
Sardines, canned in brine	3.5
Sardines, canned in oil	3.5
Sardines, canned in tomato sauce	3.5
Sardines, grilled	1.4

Unless otherwise stated, values for bottled and canned seafood are for drained weights.

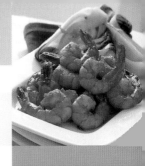

ENERGY cal	ENERGY J	FAT g	SATURATED FAT g	PROTEIN g	CARBOHYDRATE g	FIBER g
318	1318	25	Trace	27	25	Trace
636	2640	49	5.4	26	24	Trace
258	1088	4	0.5	55	Trace	0
474	1970	36	8	38	0	0
258	1070	19	4.1	20	2	Trace
438	1819	31	6.4	39	0	0
351	1461	25	5.1	31	0	0
531	2198	46	9.5	28	0	0
67	285	0	0.1	16	0	0
150	629	5	1.4	26	0	0
133	561	5	1.4	22	0	0
200	843	3	0.5	42	0	0
120	506	2	0.3	25	0	0
395	1651	24	0	11	36	Trace
639	2657	48	5.4	13	41	Trace
125	525	2	0.4	26	0	0
514	2144	34	9	30	24	1
342	1427	21	2.3	27	13	0.3
261	1094	14	1.5	21	14	0.5
121	510	2	0.4	25	0	0
129	542	3	0.7	25	0	0
369	1531	27	6.6	18	13	0.5
176	735	11	2.1	20	0	0
153	644	7	1.3	24	0	0
180	750	11	1.9	20	0	0
167	700	8	1.7	22	0	0
80	335	3	0.4	14	0	0
152	634	10	1.8	15	0	0
172	721	10	2.8	22	0	0
220	918	14	2.9	23	0	0
162	678	10	2.8	17	1	Trace
78	326	4	1.2	10	0	0

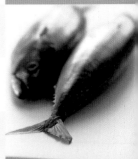

FISH & SEAFOOD

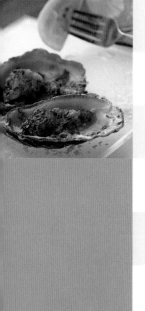

FISH	AVERAGE PORTION oz
Sea bass, broiled	3.5
Skate, grilled	7.6
Skate, in batter, fried	6
Swordfish, grilled	4.4
Trout, brown, steamed	5.5
Trout, rainbow, grilled	5.5
Tuna, canned in brine	1.6
Tuna, canned in oil	1.6
Tuna, raw	1.6
Whitebait, in flour, fried	2.8
Whiting, in crumbs, fried	2.7
Whiting, steamed	3

FISH PRODUCTS AND DISHES	
Caviar, bottled in brine	0.7
Fish cakes, fried	3.5
Fish cakes, grilled	3.5
Fish cakes, salmon, grilled	3.5
Fish fingers, cod, fried	2
Fish fingers, cod, grilled	2
Fish paste	0.4
Kedgeree	10.6
Mackerel pâté, smoked	1.4
Salmon en croûte, store bought	3.5
Taramasalata	1.6
Tuna pâté	1.4

SEAFOOD AND SHELLFISH	
Calamari, in batter, fried	4.2
Clams, breaded and fried	3
Crab, boiled, dressed with shell	4.6
Crab, canned in brine	1.4

Unless otherwise stated, values for bottled and canned seafood are for drained weights. Dishes are homemade unless otherwise stated.

ENERGY cal	ENERGY J	FAT g	SATURATED FAT g	PROTEIN g	CARBOHYDRATE g	FIBER g
125	524	3	0.7	24	0	0
170	725	1	0.2	41	0	0
286	1193	17	4.3	25	8	0.3
174	729	6	1.5	29	0	0
209	877	7	1.6	36	0	0
209	876	8	1.7	33	0	0
45	190	1	0.1	11	0	0
85	357	4	0.7	12	0	0
61	258	2	0.5	11	0	0
420	1739	38	2.1	16	4	0.2
309	1298	17	1.8	29	11	0.3
78	331	1	0.1	18	0	0
17	73	1	0.2	2	0	0
218	912	14	1.4	8	16	0.6
154	650	5	0.6	10	20	0.6
273	1137	20	2.9	10	14	0.7
133	557	8	2	7	9	0.3
112	469	5	1.6	8	9	0.4
17	71	1	0.5	2	0	0
498	2103	24	6.9	43	32	Trace
147	608	14	2.5	5	1	Trace
288	1202	19	3.1	12	18	0.3
227	935	24	1.8	1	2	Trace
94	393	7	3.1	7	0	Trace
234	978	12	2.5	14	19	0.6
172	718	9	2.3	12	9	0.3
166	696	7	0.9	25	Trace	0
31	130	0	0	7	Trace	0

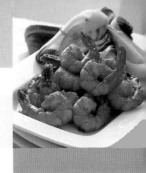

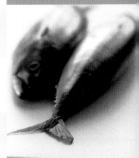

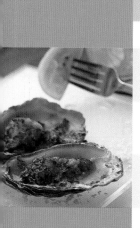

SEAFOOD AND SHELLFISH

	AVERAGE PORTION OZ
Lobster, boiled, dressed with shell	8.8
Mussels, boiled and shelled	1.4
Mussels, canned or bottled without shells	1.4
Oysters, battered or breaded, and fried	5
Oysters, uncooked and shelled	4.2
Prawns, boiled and shelled	2
Scallops, steamed and shelled	2.5
Shrimps, breaded and fried	3
Squid, fried	3

SEAFOOD PRODUCTS AND DISHES

Clam chowder, Manhattan style, canned, chunky	8.4
Clam chowder, Manhattan style, canned	8.6
Clam chowder, New England, canned	8.8
Clam and tomato juice, canned	5.8
Crabsticks	3.5
Cream of shrimp soup, canned	8.8
Scampi, in breadcrumbs, frozen, fried	6
Seafood cocktail	3.1
Seafood pasta, store bought	10.2
Shrimps, canned	3
Shrimps, imitation, made from surimi	3

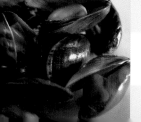

Unless otherwise stated, values for bottled and canned seafood are for drained weights. Dishes are homemade unless otherwise stated.

ENERGY cal	ENERGY J	FAT g	SATURATED FAT g	PROTEIN g	CARBOHYDRATE g	FIBER g
258	1088	4	0.5	55	Trace	0
42	176	1	0.2	7	1	0
39	166	1	0.2	7	1	0
368	1542	18	4.6	13	40	0.3
78	330	2	0.2	13	3	0
59	251	1	0.1	14	0	0
00	001	1	0.0	10	0	Trace
206	861	10	1.8	18	10	0.3
149	622	6	1.6	15	7	0
134	562	3	2.1	7	19	2.9
78	327	2	0.4	2	12	1.5
164	684	7	3	9	17	1.5
80	334	0	0.1	1	18	0.3
68	290	0	0	10	7	0
164	684	9	5.8	7	14	0.2
403	1685	23	2.4	16	35	0
77	325	1	0.3	14	3	0
319	1334	14	8.1	26	22	1.2
102	427	2	0.3	20	1	0
86	360	1	0.2	11	8	0

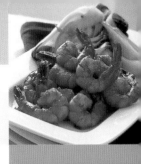

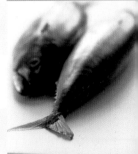

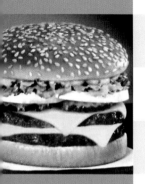

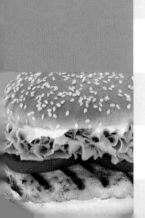

BURGER KING	AVERAGE PORTION g
Bacon Double Cheeseburger	193
BK ¼ lb. Burger™	210
BK Big Fish®	262
BK Homestyle™ Griller	242
BK Smokehouse Cheddar™ Griller	241
BK Veggie™ Burger	173
Cheeseburger	133
Chicken Tenders® (6)	92
Chicken Whopper®	272
Chicken Whopper JR.®	165
Double Cheeseburger	189
Double Hamburger	164
Double Whopper®	401
Double Whopper® with cheese	426
Egg'wich™ w/ Canadian bacon & egg	142
Egg'wich™ w/ Canadian bacon, egg & cheese	155
Egg'wich™ w/ egg & cheese	140
French Fries, large	160
French Fries, medium	117
French Fries, small	74
Hamburger	121
Hash Brown Rounds (sm)	75
King Size Fries	194
King Supreme™	196
Onion Rings, large	137
Onion Rings, medium	91
Whopper®	304
Whopper JR.®	158
Whopper JR.® with cheese	160
Whopper® with cheese	329

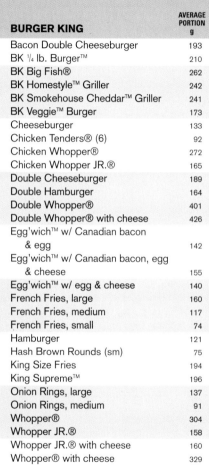

Information copyright © Burger King. All figures are for sandwiches with mayo.

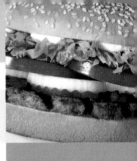

ENERGY kcal	ENERGY kJ	FAT g	SATURATED FAT g	PROTEIN g	CARBOHYDRATE g	FIBRE g
580	2331.6	34	17	35	32	2
490	1969.8	21	8	26	50	3
710	2854.2	39	15	24	66	4
480	1929.6	27	11	26	35	2
720	2894.4	48	19	39	32	2
290	1165.8	10	1.5	14	45	4
360	1477.2	17	8	19	31	2
150	1085	11	1	10	15	1
580	2331.6	26	5	39	48	3
270	1085.4	14	2.5	26	30	2
540	2170.8	31	15	32	32	2
450	1809	24	10	28	31	2
1060	4261.2	69	25	59	52	4
1150	4623	76	30	64	53	4
380	1527.6	19	4	15	35	3
420	1688.4	23	7	18	36	3
410	1648.2	23	7	15	36	3
500	2010	25	7	6	63	5
360	1447.2	18	5	4	46	4
230	924.6	11	3	3	29	2
310	1246.2	13	5	17	31	2
230	924.6	15	4	2	23	2
600	2412	30	8	7	76	6
550	2211	34	14	30	32	2
480	1929.6	23	6	7	60	5
320	1286.4	16	4	4	40	3
760	3055.2	46	14	35	52	4
390	1567.8	22	7	17	32	2
440	1768.8	26	9	19	32	2
850	3417	53	30	39	53	4

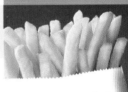

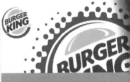

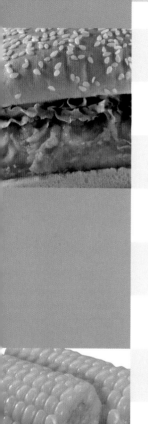

KENTUCKY FRIED CHICKEN	AVERAGE PORTION g
BBQ Baked Beans	156
Biscuit	56
Blazin Strips (3)	129
Blazin Twister	246
Cole Slaw	142
Colonel's Crispy Strips® (3)	150
Corn on the Cob	162
Extra Crispy™ Chicken – Breast	162
Extra Crispy™ Chicken – Drumstick	60
Extra Crispy™ Chicken – Thigh	114
Grean Beans	132
Honey BBQ Flavored Sandwich	178
Honey BBQ Strips (3)	178
Hot & Spicy Chicken –- Breast	179
Hot & Spicy Chicken – Drumstick	60
Hot & Spicy Chicken – Thigh	128
Hot Wings™ (6)	135
Macaroni & Cheese	153
Mashed Potatoes with Gravy	136
Original Recipe® Chicken – Breast	161
Original Recipe® Chicken – Drumstick	59
Original Recipe® Chicken – Thigh	126
Original Recipe® Sandwich with Sauce	200
Popcorn Chicken, large	170
Popcorn Chicken, small	99
Potato Salad	160
Spicy Crispy Strips (3)	115
Tender Roast® Sandwich with Sauce	211
Triple Crunch® Sandwich with Sauce	189
Triple Crunch® Zinger Sandwich with Sauce	210
Twister®	240

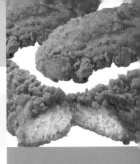

ENERGY kcal	ENERGY kJ	FAT g	SATURATED FAT g	PROTEIN g	CARBOHYDRATE g	FIBRE g
190	763.8	25	1	6	33	6
180	723.6	80	2.5	4	20	<1
315	1266.3§	16	4	26	21	1
719	2890.4	43	12	30	56	4
232	932.64	121	2	2	26	3
340	1366.8	16	4.5	28	20	0
150	603	15	0	5	35	2
170	1889.1	28	8	34	19	0
160	643.2	10	2.5	12	5	0
370	1487.4	26	7	21	12	0
45	180.9	15	0.5	1	7	3
310	1246.2	6	2	28	37	2
377	1515.5	15	4	27	33	4
450	1809	27	8	33	20	0
140	562.8	9	2.5	13	4	0
390	1567.8	28	8	22	14	0
471	1893.4	33	8	27	18	2
180	723.6	70	3	7	21	2
120	482.4	50	1	1	17	2
370	1487.4	19	6	40	11	0
140	562.8	8	2	14	4	0
360	1447.2	25	7	22	12	0
450	1809	22	5	29	33	2
60	2492.4	40	10	30	36	0
362	1455.2	23	6	17	21	0.2
230	924.6	130	2	4	23	3
335	1346.7	15	4	25	23	<1
350	1407	15	3	32	26	1
490	1969.8	29	6	28	39	2
550	2211	32	7	28	39	2
600	2412	34	7	22	52	4

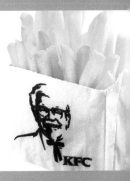

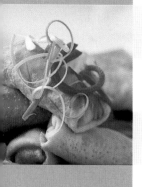

BURGERS

	AVERAGE PORTION OZ
Cheeseburger, large, double patty	9.1
Cheeseburger, large, single patty	7.7
Cheeseburger, regular, double patty	8
Cheeseburger, triple patty, plain	10.6
Hamburger, large, double patty	7.9
Hamburger, large, single patty, with condiments	6.1
Hamburger, large, triple patty, with condiments	9.2
Hamburger, regular, double patty, plain	6.2
Hamburger, regular, double patty, with condiments	7.6
Hamburger, regular, single patty, plain	3.2
Hamburger, regular, single patty, with condiments	3.8

PIZZAS

Cheese and tomato, deep pan, store bought	7.8
Cheese and tomato, deep pan	7.8
Cheese and tomato, French bread, frozen, store bought	7
Cheese and tomato, frozen, store bought	7
Cheese and tomato, thin base	4.1
Chicken, deep pan, store bought	8.1
Ham and pineapple, store bought	7
Meat, deep pan	8.1
Meat topped, frozen, store bought	7
meat topped, thin base	5.3
Meat, deep pan, store bought	8.1
Vegetable, deep pan	10.2
Pizza, vegetable, thin base	5.3

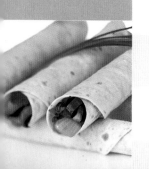

Unless otherwise stated, burgers include condiments and vegetables and pizzas are takeout.

ENERGY cal	ENERGY J	FAT g	SATURATED FAT g	PROTEIN g	CARBOHYDRATE g	FIBER g
704	2946	44	17.7	38	40	2.1
563	2354	33	15	28	38	2.1
650	2718	35	12.8	30	53	2.1
796	3332	51	21.7	56	27	2.1
540	2260	27	10.5	34	40	2.1
427	1785	21	7.9	23	37	2.1
692	2893	41	15.9	50	29	2.1
544	2276	28	10.4	30	43	2
576	2410	32	12	32	39	2.1
274	1148	12	4.1	12	31	2
272	1140	10	3.6	12	34	2.3
471	1987	15	7.7	24	64	4.8
547	2310	16	11.4	27	77	4.8
461	1942	16	6.6	21	63	3.8
475	2002	18	9	23	60	3.8
322	1355	12	9.3	17	39	2.2
565	2382	19	7.8	31	72	4.8
521	2196	17	6.8	27	69	4.8
557	2345	21	14	30	67	4.6
496	2087	19	7.6	23	61	3.8
391	1642	18	7.5	21	39	2.8
624	2624	25	9.7	32	73	4.8
621	2624	18	7.8	32	88	4.9
332	1398	11	4.1	16	44	2.8

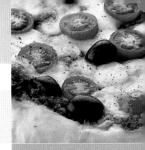

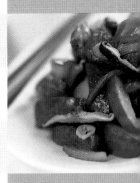

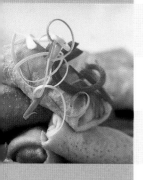

MEXICAN DISHES

	AVERAGE PORTION oz
Burrito, beans	7.6
Burrito, beans and cheese	6.5
Burrito, beans and chili peppers	7.1
Burrito, beans and meat	8
Burrito, beans, cheese, and beef	7.1
Burrito, beef	7.6
Burrito, beef and chili peppers	7
Burrito, beef, cheese, and chili peppers	10.6
Chimichanga, beef	6.1
Chimichanga, beef and cheese	6.4
Chimichanga, beef and chili peppers	6.7
Chimichanga, beef, cheese, and chili peppers	6.3
Enchilada, cheese	5.7
Enchilada, cheese and beef	6.7
Enchilada, vegetable	12.7
Fajita, chicken, meat only	6
Nachos, cheese	6
Nachos, cheese and jalapeno peppers	7.1
Nachos, cheese, beans, ground beef, and peppers	9
Tostada, beans and cheese	5.1
Tostada, beans, beef, and cheese	7.9
Tostada, beef and cheese	5.7

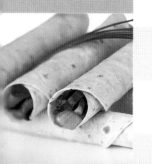

MISCELLANEOUS

Corndog	6.1
Hotdog, plain	3.4
Hotdog, with chili	4
Hush puppies	2.7
Pancakes with butter and syrup	8.1

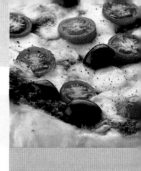

ENERGY cal	ENERGY J	FAT g	SATURATED FAT g	PROTEIN g	CARBOHYDRATE g	FIBER g
447	1871	13	6.9	14	71	1.5
378	1579	12	6.8	15	55	1.5
412	1724	15	7.6	16	58	1.5
508	2125	18	8.3	22	66	1.5
331	1384	13	7.1	15	40	1.5
524	2191	21	10.5	27	59	1.5
426	1783	17	8	22	49	1.5
632	2645	25	10.4	41	64	1.5
425	1777	20	8.5	20	43	1.5
443	1854	23	11.2	20	39	1.5
424	1773	19	8.3	18	46	1.5
364	1521	18	8.4	15	38	1.5
319	1337	19	10.6	10	29	1
323	1350	18	9	12	30	1
525	1690	26	7.6	23	54	7.6
213	676	11	3.6	29	1	1.7
438	1208	31	11.6	18	24	3.4
608	2544	34	14	17	60	2
569	2379	31	12.5	20	56	2
223	935	10	5.4	10	27	1.5
333	1393	17	11.5	16	30	1.5
315	1317	16	10.4	19	23	1.5
460	1925	19	5.2	17	56	1
242	1012	15	5.1	10	18	1
296	1240	13	4.9	14	31	1
257	1074	12	2.7	5	35	1.5
520	2174	14	5.9	8	91	1

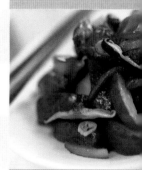

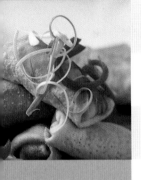

INDIAN DISHES

	AVERAGE PORTION oz
Chicken biryani	14
Chicken dhansak	12.3
Chicken jalfrezi	12.3
Chicken korma	12.3
Chicken tikka	12.3
Lamb balti	12.3
Lamb rogan josh	12.3
Poppadoms	2.5
Samosa, meat	2.5
Vegetable balti	12.3
Vegetable biryani	12.3

ASIAN DISHES

Aromatic crispy duck	4.4
Chicken chop suey	15.9
Chicken chow mein	12.3
Chicken fried rice	12.3
Chicken satay	6
Chicken with cashew nuts	12.7
Egg fried rice	9.5
Green chicken curry	12.3
Meat spring roll	1.9
Sesame shrimp toasts	2.5
Shrimp crackers	2.5
Spare ribs	12
Stir-fried beef with green peppers in black bean sauce	12.7
Stir-fried Thai vegetable curry	12.3
Stir-fried vegetables	12
Sweet and sour chicken	10.6
Szechuan prawns with vegetables	12.3

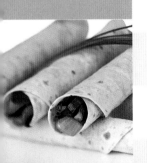

ENERGY cal	ENERGY J	FAT g	SATURATED FAT g	PROTEIN g	CARBOHYDRATE g	FIBER g
651	2144	30	8.0	34	66	4.4
503	1509	30	6.0	40	21	6.7
416	1203	27	5.3	34	11	7.0
668	1753	51	20.0	44	8	7.0
421	1470	15	5.6	71	Trace	1.0
534	1518	35	8.8	43	11	6.7
510	1422	35	9.8	43	6	3.1
361	916	27	5.6	8	20	4.1
191	553	12	3.2	8	13	1.5
373	983	28	5.3	8	23	7.7
467	1468	25	4.9	10	55	6.0
412	1107	30	9.1	35	15	1.1
363	1095	21	3.6	37	7	5.4
516	1662	25	4.2	30	46	3.9
562	1948	21	3.5	23	75	0.0
324	1006	18	4.9	37	5	3.7
470	1331	31	5.4	38	10	0.0
491	1809	13	1.6	12	87	2.2
417	1125	30	18.2	31	5	8.4
133	374	9	2.1	4	10	1.0
268	699	21	2.7	9	12	1.3
386	1061	27	2.6	0	37	0.8
873	2358	64	10.2	75	7	1.0
373	1158	20	5.0	38	11	6.5
351	882	29	13.7	13	11	9.1
177	455	14	2.4	6	7	6.1
575	1810	30	3.9	23	57	1.8
297	912	16	1.8	27	11	4.9

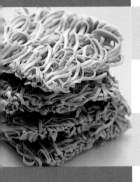

RICE, PASTA AND NOODLES	AVERAGE PORTION OZ
Brown rice, boiled	6.3
Macaroni, boiled	8.1
Macaroni, wholewheat, boiled	8.1
Noodles, egg, boiled	8.1
Noodles, boiled	8.1
Noodles, fried	8.1
Red rice, boiled	8.1
Savory rice, cooked	6.3
Spaghetti, boiled	7.8
Spaghetti, wholewheat, boiled	8.1
White rice, easy cook, boiled	6.3
White rice, fried in lard/drippings	10.6
White rice, glutinous, boiled	8.1
White rice, polished, boiled	8.1

RICE AND PASTA DISHES

Budget Gourmet Italian sausage lasagna, frozen	10.5
Cannelloni, meat, store bought	9.2
Cannelloni, spinach	12
Cannelloni, vegetable	12
Chef Boyardee beef ravioli in tomato and meat sauce, canned	8.5
Chef Boyardee mini beef ravioli in tomato and meat sauce, canned	8.8
Chef Boyardee Spaghetti & Meatballs in Tomato Sauce, canned entrée	240
Chicken risotto	12
Healthy Choice Spaghetti with meat sauce, frozen entrée	283
Lasagne, meat, store bought	14.8
Lasagne, spinach	14.8
Lasagne, spinach, wholewheat	14.8

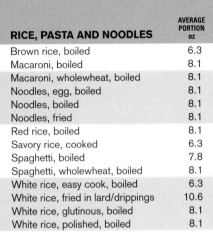

Unless otherwise stated, all dishes are homemade.

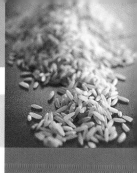

ENERGY cal	ENERGY J	FAT g	SATURATED FAT g	PROTEIN g	CARBOHYDRATE g	FIBER g
254	1075	2	0.5	5	58	1.4
198	840	1	0.2	7	43	2.1
198	840	1	0.2	7	43	6.4
143	607	1	0.2	5	30	1.4
143	607	1	0.2	6	30	1.6
352	1467	26	1	4	26	1.2
184	784	1	0.2	4	43	1.4
256	1078	6	2	5	47	2.5
229	972	2	0.2	8	49	2.6
260	1116	2	0.2	11	53	8.1
248	1057	2	0.5	5	56	0.2
393	1662	10	4.2	7	75	1.8
150	633	1	0.2	4	34	0.5
283	1201	1	0.2	5	68	0.5
456	1907	24	8.2	21	40	3
315	1326	13	5.2	17	35	3.1
449	1880	26	7.8	15	43	2.7
493	2067	31	11.6	15	43	2.4
229	959	5	2.5	8	37	3.7
239	1000	5	1.8	9	41	3.3
250	1044	9	3.9	9	34	2.2
546	2310	10	4.5	31	84	Trace
255	1067	3	1	14	43	5.1
601	2533	26	11.8	31	66	2.9
365	1541	13	5.5	15	53	4.6
391	1659	13	5.5	18	55	9.7

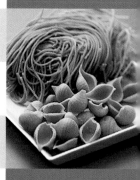

RICE, PASTA
& NOODLES

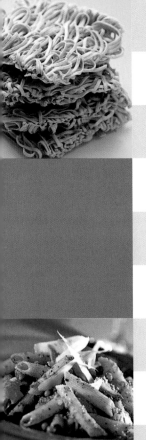

RICE AND PASTA DISHES	AVERAGE PORTION oz
Lasagne, vegetable	14.8
Lasagne, vegetable, wholewheat	14.8
Michelina's Spaghetti with Meatballs & Pomodoro Sauce, Low Fat frozen entrée	
Pasta with ham and mushroom sauce	8.3
Pasta with meat and tomato sauce	8.3
Peppers, stuffed with rice	6.2
Pilaff, mushroom	6.3
Pilaff, vegetable	180
Ravioli, stuffed with cheese, tomato and herbs, store bought	250
Ravioli, stuffed with meat and vegetables, store bought	8.8
Rice and blackeye beans	7
Rice and blackeye beans, brown rice	7
Risotto, chicken	12
Risotto, vegetable, brown rice	10.2
Risotto, vegetable	10.2
Spaghetti and meat sauce, store bought	14
Stouffer's lasagna with meat and sauce, frozen	7.6
Stouffer's Lean Cuisine spaghetti with meat sauce, frozen 326	313
Stouffer's Lean Cuisine spaghetti with meatballs and sauce, frozen 269	299
Tortellini, stuffed with cheese and ham, store bought	8.8
Vine leaves, stuffed with rice	2.8

Unless otherwise stated, all dishes are homemade.

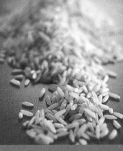

ENERGY cal	ENERGY J	FAT g	SATURATED FAT g	PROTEIN g	CARBOHYDRATE g	FIBER g
428	1810	18	9.2	17	52	4.2
445	1877	19	9.2	20	52	8.8
284	312	1306	7	2.2	14	49 6.2
284	1194	14	8.2	13	27	2.1
263	1102	10	4	16	30	2
149	630	4	0.7	3	27	2.3
248	1048	8	1.5	4	43	0.7
248	1053	8	4.3	5	43	1
304	1267	13	7.9	17	30	0.6
324	1350	15	8.9	16	34	3.4
366	1556	7	3	12	68	2.8
350	1488	7	3	11	66	3.6
546	2310	10	4.5	31	84	Trace
415	1749	19	2.6	12	54	7
426	1798	19	2.9	12	56	6.4
432	1816	23	9.2	37	21	3.6
277	1161	11	4.7	19	26	3.2
	1311	6	1.4	14	51	5.5
	1248	8	2.1	18	40	4.6
316	1318	9	6	16	44	1.4
210	875	14	2.1	2	19	1.0

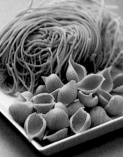

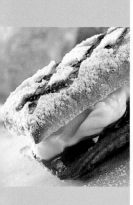

BREAD AND CAKES	AVERAGE PORTION oz
Banana bread, homemade	3
Brioche	1.6
Brown bread, sliced	1.3
Brown rolls	1.7
Campione d'Italia garlic bread, frozen	1
Carrot cake, homemade, un-iced	3
Cheese-topped rolls, white	3
Chocolate cake	1.4
Chocolate cake, with butter icing	2.2
Chocolate fudge cake	3.4
Ciabatta, plain	1.8
Cinnamon-raisin loaf	1.2
Coconut cake	1.4
Cornbread, made with low-fat (2%) milk	2.3
Doughnuts, cake-type, chocolate, sugared or glazed	1.5
Doughnuts, cake-type, plain	1.7
Doughnuts, cake-type, plain, chocolate-coated or frosted	1.5
Doughnuts, cake-type, plain, sugared or glazed	1.6
Doughnuts, cake-type, wheat, sugared or glazed	1.9
Doughnuts, french crullers, glazed	1.5
Doughnuts, yeast-leavened, glazed	2
Doughnuts, yeast-leavened, creme-filled	3
Doughnuts, yeast-leavened, jelly-filled	3
Focaccia, herb/garlic and coriander	1.8
French baguette, white	1.4
French baguette, white, part baked	1.4
French loaf, multigrain	1.4
French ficelle, white	1.4
French/Vienna bread	1
French/Vienna bread, toasted	1

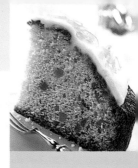

ENERGY cal	ENERGY J	FAT g	SATURATED FAT g	PROTEIN g	CARBOHYDRATE g	FIBER g
230	968	9	5.6	4	35	1.5
144	607	4	2.8	4	24	1.0
75	317	1	0.2	3	15	1.3
113	482	2	0.3	5	22	1.8
101	424	5	0.8	2	12	1.3
349	1454	25	6.4	5	28	2.1
241	1016	7	3.4	9	38	1.2
182	763	11	8.2	3	20	0.5
313	1306	19	14.3	4	33	0.8
351	1479	14	4.5	5	55	0.9
135	574	2	0.3	5	26	1.2
18	76	1	0.2	3	0	0.9
174	726	10	2.6	3	20	1
173	723	5	1	4	28	1
175	733	8	2.2	2	24	0.9
198	828	11	1.7	2	23	0.7
204	853	13	3.5	2	21	0.9
192	802	10	2.7	2	23	0.7
194	813	10	1.6	3	23	1.2
169	707	8	1.9	1	24	0.5
226	944	13	3.3	4	25	0.7
307	1284	21	4.6	5	26	0.7
289	1210	16	4.1	5	33	0.7
147	620	4	0.6	5	26	0.7
109	465	1	0.1	4	24	1.0
108	458	1	0.1	4	23	1.0
110	467	1	0.1	4	22	1.0
101	431	1	0.1	4	21	1.0
77	321	1	0.2	2	15	0.8
86	362	1	0.2	3	16	1

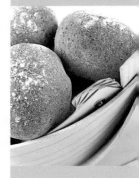

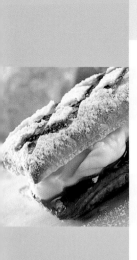

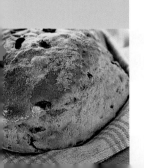

BREAD AND CAKES	AVERAGE PORTION oz
Frosted cupcakes	1
Fruit cake, plain	2
Fruit cake, rich	2.5
Fruit cake, wholemeal	3.2
Garlic bread	0.7
Gingerbread	1.8
Jelly roll	1
Italian bread	1
Light white bread, sliced	0.7
Muffins, blueberry, homemade with low fat (2%) milk	2
Muffins, blueberry, store-bought	2
Muffins, blueberry, toasting, toasted	1.1
Muffins, corn, homemade with low fat (2%) milk	2
Muffins, corn, store-bought	2
Muffins, corn, toasting, toasted	1.3
Muffins, English, multigrain	2.3
Muffins, English, plain, enriched	2
Muffins, English, plain, unenriched	2
Muffins, English, raisin-cinnamon/ apple-cinnamon	2
Muffins, English, wheat	2
Muffins, English, wholewheat	2.3
Muffins, oatbran	2
Muffins, plain, homemade with low fat (2%) milk	2
Muffins, wheatbran with raisins, toasting, toasted	1.2
Multigrain bread, sliced	1.3
Multigrain rolls	56
Naan bread, garlic and coriander/plain	5.6
Oatmeal bread	1
Oatmeal bread, reduced-calorie	0.7

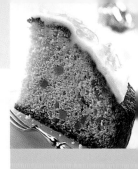

ENERGY cal	ENERGY J	FAT g	SATURATED FAT g	PROTEIN g	CARBOHYDRATE g	FIBER g
122	515	3	2.8	1	21	0.4
212	894	9	3.5	3	35	1.6
239	1007	8	2.4	3	42	1.2
327	1373	14	4.3	5	48	2.2
73	306	4	1.9	2	9	1.0
190	799	6	1.9	3	32	0.6
83	352	1	0.3	2	17	0.2
76	318	1	0.2	2	14	0.8
46	193	1	0.1	2	9	0.5
162	679	6	1.2	4	23	1.5
158	661	4	0.8	3	27	1.5
103	432	3	0.5	2	18	0.6
180	754	7	1.3	4	25	1.9
174	727	5	0.8	3	29	1.9
114	478	4	0.6	2	19	0.5
155	649	1	0.2	6	31	1.8
134	560	1	0.1	4	26	1.5
134	560	1	0.1	4	26	1.5
139	580	2	0.2	4	28	1.7
127	532	1	0.2	5	26	2.6
134	560	1	0.2	6	27	4.4
154	644	4	0.6	4	28	2.6
169	706	6	1.2	4	24	1.5
106	445	3	0.5	2	19	2.8
87	369	1	0.3	4	18	1.3
133	565	2	0.3	6	24	2.0
456	1929	12	1.6	12	80	3.2
73	304	1	0.2	2	13	1.1
48	202	1	0.1	2	10	1.1

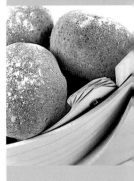

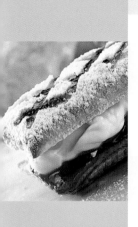

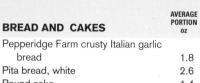

BREAD AND CAKES	AVERAGE PORTION oz
Pepperidge Farm crusty Italian garlic bread	1.8
Pita bread, white	2.6
Pound cake	1.4
Pumpernickel bread	1.1
Rolls, hamburger or hotdog, multigrain	1.5
Rolls, hamburger or hotdog, plain	1.5
Rolls, hamburger or hotdog, reduced-calorie	1.5
Sandwich bread, white	0.5
Scones, cheese	1.7
Scones, fruit	1.7
Scones, plain	1.7
Scones, wholewheat	1.8
Scones, wholewheat, fruit	1.8
Sponge cake, fat-free	2
Sponge cake, frozen	2
Sponge cake, with buttercream frosting	2
Strawberry tartlets	1.8
Swiss cake rolls, chocolate, individual	1
Tortilla, wheat, soft	5.6
Waffles	2.2
Wheatgerm bread	1
White bread, crusty bloomer	1.2
White bread, farmhouse, large	1.2
White bread, farmhouse, small	0.9
White bread, premium	1.2
White bread, standard	1.2
White bread, standard, toasted	1.2
White rolls, crusty	1.8
White rolls, soft	1.6
Wholewheat bread	1.3
Wholewheat bread, toasted	1.3
Wholewheat rolls	1.7

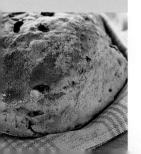

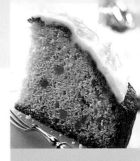

ENERGY cal	ENERGY J	FAT g	SATURATED FAT g	PROTEIN g	CARBOHYDRATE g	FIBER g
186	779	10	2.4	4	21	1.3
191	813	1	0.7	7	41	1.8
157	661	6	3.5	2	23	0.4
67	283	1	0.1	2	15	2.1
113	473	3	0.6	4	19	1.6
123	515	2	0.5	4	22	1.2
84	353	1	0.1	4	18	2.7
36	153	1	0.2	1	7	0.3
174	731	9	4.9	5	21	0.8
152	640	5	1.6	4	25	0.8
174	731	7	2.4	3	26	0.9
163	684	7	2.4	4	22	2.6
162	683	6	2	4	24	2.5
171	722	4	1	6	31	0.5
190	795	10	3.1	2	24	0.4
294	1228	18	5.6	3	31	0.4
111	466	6	3.2	1	14	0.6
101	426	5	1.4	1	17	0.3
451	1903	14	2.9	12	73	3.0
217	911	11	4.7	6	26	1
66	281	1	0.2	3	12	1.2
86	368	1	0.2	3	18	0.8
83	353	1	0.2	3	17	0.7
66	281	1	0.2	2	14	0.7
83	352	1	0.2	3	17	0.7
79	335	1	0.1	3	17	0.7
97	414	1	0.1	3	21	0.0
131	558	1	0.3	5	27	1.2
114	485	1	0.3	4	23	0.9
82	349	1	0.2	4	16	1.9
102	431	1	0.2	5	20	0.0
117	498	2	0.2	5	22	2.1

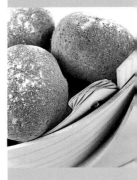

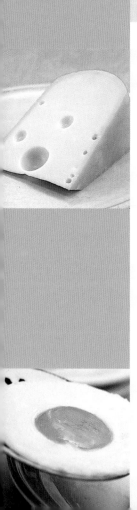

CHEESE	AVERAGE PORTION oz
Brie, without rind	1.4
Camembert	1.4
Cheddar, English, white	1.4
Cheddar, half-fat (15% fat)	1.4
Cheddar, vegetarian	1.4
Cheese spread	1
Cheshire, white	1.4
Cottage (4% fat)	1.4
Cottage, low-fat (1.5–2% fat)	1.4
Danish Blue	1
Dolcelatte, without rind	1.4
Double Gloucester	1.4
Edam	1.4
Emmental	1.4
Fontina	0.9
Fromage frais, fruit	3.5
Fromage frais, fruit, virtually fat-free	3.5
Fromage frais, natural	3.5
Fromage frais, natural, virtually fat-free	3.5
Goat	1.9
Gouda	1.4
Halloumi	1.4
Lancashire	1.4
Mascarpone	1.9
Monterey Jack	0.9
Mozzarella, fresh	1.9
Mozzarella, grated	1.9
Paneer	1.4
Parmesan, drums, freshly grated	0.7
Parmesan, wedges, freshly grated	0.7
Pecorino	0.9
Port Salut	1.4
Processed cheese, slices	0.7
Provolone	0.9

Unless otherwise specified, generic cheeses are made with cow's milk.

ENERGY cal	ENERGY J	FAT g	SATURATED FAT g	PROTEIN g	CARBOHYDRATE g	FIBER g
144	596	12	7.3	8	2	0
116	482	9	6.0	9	Trace	0
166	690	14	8.7	10	0	0
109	456	6	4.3	13	Trace	0
156	647	13	8.3	10	Trace	0
81	335	7	4.7	3	2	0
152	630	13	8.5	9	Trace	0
36	149	2	0.9	5	0	0
28	118	1	0.4	5	0	0
103	425	9	5.7	6	Trace	0
158	652	14	8.7	7	Trace	0
165	684	14	9.3	10	Trace	0
136	566	10	6.3	11	Trace	0
160	663	12	8.2	12	Trace	0
110	462	9	5.4	7	0	0
135	566	5.6	0.0	5.2	16.9	0.4
50	211	0.2	0.0	6.7	5.6	0.4
113	468	8.0	5.6	6.0	4.4	Trace
48	205	0.1	0.0	7.5	4.6	Trace
174	722	14	9.8	12	Trace	0
151	625	12	8.1	10	Trace	0
124	516	9	6.6	10	0	0
153	633	13	8.4	10	Trace	0
230	949	24	16.2	3	Trace	0
107	443	30	5.4	25	0	0
141	587	11	7.6	10	Trace	0
164	680	12	8.1	14	Trace	0
130	539	10	6.2	10	Trace	0
97	403	7	4.6	9	Trace	0
82	343	6	3.9	7	Trace	0
110	459	8	4.8	1	1	0
133	554	10	7.2	10	Trace	0
59	244	5	2.8	4	1	0
99	417	8	4.8	7	1	0

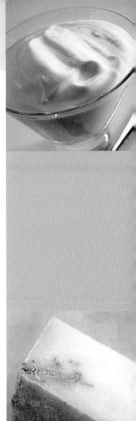

CHEESE

	AVERAGE PORTION oz
Red Leceister	1.4
Ricotta	1.9
Romano	0.9
Roquefort	0.9
Soft white spreadable, low-fat (<10%)	1
Soft white spreadable, reduced-fat (15%)	1
Soft white spreadable, full-fat	1
St. Paulin	1.4
Stilton, blue	1.2
Wensleydale	1.4

CREAM AND SUBSTITUTES

Cream, clotted	1.6
Cream, heavy	1
Cream, light	0.5
Cream, sour	1
Cream, whipping	1
Cream, frozen, whipping	1
Cream, sterilized, canned	1.6
Cream, UHT, canned spray	0.4
Cream, UHT, half-and-half	0.5
Cream, UHT, light	15
Cream, UHT, whipping	1
Crème fraîche	1.2
Crème fraîche, low-fat	1.2
Half-and-half	1
Non-dairy, whipping	1

Unless otherwise specified, generic cheeses are made with cow's milk and cream is fresh.

ENERGY cal	ENERGY J	FAT g	SATURATED FAT g	PROTEIN g	CARBOHYDRATE g	FIBER g
161	667	13	8.9	10	Trace	0
79	329	6	3.8	5	1	0
110	459	8	4.8	1	1	0
105	438	9	5.4	6	1	0
43	182	2	1.7	4	1	0
56	231	5	3.4	3	Trace	0
94	306	9	6.7	2	Trace	0
133	554	10	7.2	10	Trace	0
143	594	12	8.1	8	Trace	0
152	632	13	8.5	9	Trace	0
264	1086	29	17.9	1	1	0
135	555	16	9	1	1	0
30	123	3	1.8	0	1	0
62	254	6	3.8	1	1	0
112	462	12	7.4	1	1	0
114	468	12	7.5	1	1	0
108	443	11	6.7	1	2	0
31	127	2	2	0	0	0
21	86	2	1.2	0	1	0
29	122	3	1.8	0	1	0
112	462	12	7.4	1	1	0
190	792	20	13.2	1.2	1.4	0
85	355	7.5	4.5	1.8	2.5	0
44	184	4	2.5	1	1	0
96	395	9	8.4	1	1	0

EGGS

	AVERAGE PORTION OZ
Raw	2
Boiled	1.8
Duck, boiled and salted	2.5
Duck, raw	2.5
Egg yolk, raw	0.6
Free-range, raw	2
Fried in vegetable oil	2
Fried, without fat	1.8
Poached	1.8
Quail, raw	1.4

EGG DISHES

Omelette, cheese	5.3
Omelette, plain (two-egg)	4.2
Omelette, potato (two-egg)	5.3
Scrambled, with milk (two-egg)	4.2
Scrambled, without milk (two-egg)	3.5

MILK AND MILK SUBSTITUTES

Coffee creamer	0.1
Condensed milk, skim, sweetened	0.5
Condensed milk, whole, sweetened	0.5
Evaporated milk, reduced-fat	0.5
Evaporated milk, whole	0.5
Flavored milk	7.5
Goats' milk, pasteurized	5.2
Low-fat milk, pasteurized	5.2
Low-fat milk, UHT	5.2
Sheep's milk	5.2
Skim milk, dried	0.1
Skim milk, dried, with vegetable fat	0.1
Skim milk, pasteurized	5.2

Unless otherwise specified, figures are for one egg, chicken's eggs are medium-sized and milk is cow's milk.

ENERGY cal	ENERGY J	FAT g	SATURATED FAT g	PROTEIN g	CARBOHYDRATE g	FIBER g
88	367	1.9	6	8	Trace	0
74	306	1.5	5	6	Trace	0
139	575	2.7	11	10	Trace	0
122	510	2.2	9	11	Trace	0
61	252	1.6	5	3	Trace	0
86	358	1.7	7	7	Trace	0
107	447	2.4	8	8	Trace	0
87	363	1.8	6	6	Trace	0
74	306	1.5	5	6	Trace	0
60	252	1.2	4	5	Trace	0
399	1659	18.3	34	24	Trace	0
229	950	8.9	20	13	Trace	0
180	752	2.4	12	9	9	2.1
296	1230	13.9	27	13	1	0
160	664	3.3	12	14	Trace	0
16	68	1	1	0	2	0
40	171	0	0	2	9	0
50	211	2	0.9	1	8	0
18	77	1	0.2	1	2	0
23	94	1	0.9	1	1	0
146	614	3	1.9	8	23	0
88	369	5	3.4	5	6	0
67	285	2	1.5	5	7	0
67	283	2	1.6	5	7	0
139	578	8	5.5	8	7	0
10	44	0	0	1	2	0
15	61	1	0.5	1	1	0
48	204	1	0.1	5	7	0

DAIRY
PRODUCTS 91

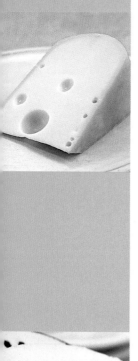

MILK AND MILK SUBSTITUTES	AVERAGE PORTION oz
Skim milk, sterilized	4.8
Skim milk, UHT	5.2
Soy milk	5.2
Soy milk, flavored	5.2
Whole milk, dried	0.1
Whole milk, pasteurized	5.2
Whole milk, sterilized	5.2
Whole milk, UHT	5.2

YOGURTS

Crème fraîche (see under cream)	
Fromage frais (see under cheese)	
Drinking yogurt	7
Probiotic yogurt drink, orange	3.5
Probiotic yogurt drink, plain	3.5
Yogurt, French set, fruit, low-fat	4.4
Yogurt, fruit	4.4
Yogurt, fruit, low-fat	4.4
Yogurt, fruit, virtually fat-free	4.4
Yogurt, Greek-style, fruit, whole milk	5.3
Yogurt, Greek-style, honey, whole milk	5.3
Yogurt, Greek-style, natural, whole milk	5.3
Yogurt, hazelnut, low-fat	4.4
Yogurt, long life, fruit, whole milk	4.4
Yogurt, natural, low-fat	4.4
Yogurt, natural, virtually fat-free	4.4
Yogurt, soy, fruit	4.4
Yogurt, toffee, low-fat	4.4
Yogurt, twin pot, fruit, virtually fat-free	4.8
Yogurt, vanilla, low-fat	4.4

Unless otherwise specified, milk is cow's milk.

ENERGY cal	ENERGY J	FAT g	SATURATED FAT g	PROTEIN g	CARBOHYDRATE g	FIBER g
44	188	1	0.1	5	7	0
47	200	1	0.1	5	7	0
47	193	2	0.4	4	1	Trace
58	245	2	0.3	4	5	Trace
15	62	1	0.5	1	1	0
96	402	6	3.5	5	7	0
96	404	6	3.5	5	7	0
96	402	6	3.5	5	7	0
124	526	Trace	Trace	6	26	Trace
67	279	0.9	0.6	1.5	13.4	1.3
68	284	1	0.7	1.7	13.1	1.4
103	435	1.4	1.0	4.3	19.5	0.3
133	564	3.8	2.5	4.9	21.4	0.3
97	412	1.4	0.9	5.1	17.1	0.3
75	318	0.5	0.0	5.9	12.5	0.3
205	857	12.6	8.4	7.2	16.8	Trace
221	927	12.5	8.4	7.7	21.0	Trace
198	824	15.3	10.2	8.4	7.2	Trace
111	469	1.9	0.8	5.5	19.1	0.3
125	529	4.3	0.0	3.9	19.1	0.3
69	294	1.3	0.9	5.9	9.3	Trace
67	286	0.3	0.0	6.6	10.3	Trace
92	388	2.3	0.3	2.9	16.0	0.4
114	484	1.1	0.8	4.8	22.6	Trace
55	236	0.1	0.1	4.5	9.7	0.7
114	484	1.1	0.8	4.8	22.6	Trace

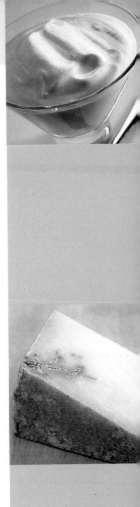

DAIRY
PRODUCTS 93

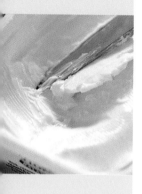

	AVERAGE PORTION oz
FATS	
Butter	
Butter	0.7
Ghee	0.25
Margarine	
Hard, animal and vegetable fats	0.4
Hard, vegetable fats	0.4
Soft, animal and vegetable fat	0.25
Soft, polyunsaturated	0.25
Other fats	
Compound cooking fat	0.5
Compound cooking fat, polyunsaturated	0.5
Dripping, beef	0.5
Ghee, vegetable	0.25
Lard	0.5
Spreads	
Blended 70% fat	0.25
Blended 40% fat	0.25
20–25% fat, not polyunsaturated	0.25
20–25% fat	0.25
35–40% fat	0.25
40% fat, not polyunsaturated	0.25
5% fat	0.25
60% fat	0.25
60% fat, with olive oil	0.25
70% fat	0.25
OILS	
Canola oil	0.4
Corn oil	0.5
Grapeseed oil	0.4
Hazelnut oil	0.1
Olive oil	0.4

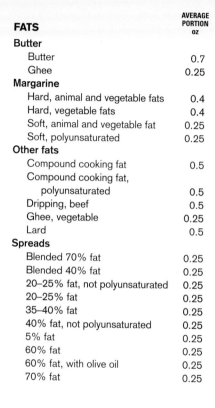

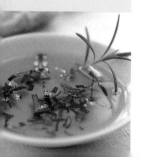

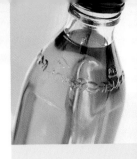

ENERGY cal	ENERGY J	FAT g	SATURATED FAT g	PROTEIN g	CARBOHYDRATE g	FIBER g
147	606	16	11	0	Trace	0
63	259	7	4.6	Trace	Trace	0
72	295	8	3.5	0	0	0
74	304	8	3.6	0	0	0
52	213	6	1.9	0	0	0
52	215	6	1.2	Trace	0	0
135	554	15	7.4	Trace	0	0
135	554	15	3.1	Trace	Trace	0
134	549	15	7.9	Trace	Trace	0
63	257	7	3.4	Trace	Trace	0
134	549	15	6	Trace	0	0
48	196	5	1.8	0	0	0
27	113	3	1.3	0	0	0
17	71	2	0.4	0	0	0
13	53	1	0.3	0	0	0
26	105	3	0.6	0	0	0
28	113	3	0.8	0	0	0
7	30	1	0.1	0	1	0.4
39	159	4	0.8	0	0	0
40	164	4	0.8	0	0	0
44	183	5	0.9	0	0	0
99	407	11	0.7	Trace	0	0
135	554	15	2.2	Trace	0	0
99	407	11	1.2	Trace	0	0
99	407	11	0.9	Trace	0	0
99	407	11	1.6	Trace	0	0

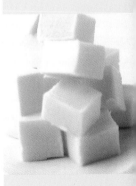

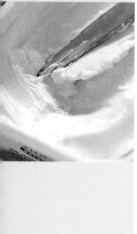

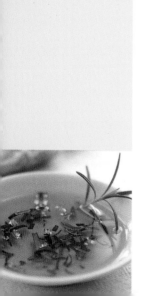

OILS

	AVERAGE PORTION oz
Palm oil	0.4
Peanut oil	0.4
Safflower oil	0.4
Sesame oil	0.1
Soya oil	0.4
Sunflower oil	0.4
Vegetable oil	0.4
Walnut oil	0.4
Wheatgerm oil	0.4

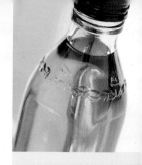

ENERGY cal	ENERGY J	FAT g	SATURATED FAT g	PROTEIN g	CARBOHYDRATE g	FIBER g
99	407	11	5.3	Trace	0	0
99	407	11	2.2	Trace	0	0
99	407	11	1.1	Trace	0	0
27	111	3	0.4	Trace	0	0
99	407	11	1.7	Trace	0	0
99	407	11	1.3	Trace	0	0
99	407	11	1.1	Trace	0	0
99	407	11	1	Trace	0	0
99	407	11	2	Trace	0	0

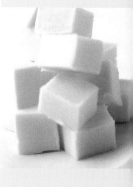

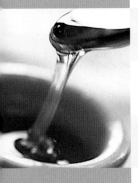

SWEET SPREADS	AVERAGE PORTION OZ
Chocolate spread	0.6
Fruit spread	0.6
Honey	0.6
Lemon curd	0.5

SAVORY SPREADS AND PATES	
Fish paste	0.4
Mackerel pâté, smoked	1.4
Meat spread	0.4
Liver sausage	1.4
Pâté, liver, tubed	1.4
Peanut butter, smooth	0.9
Peanut butter, crunchy	0.9
Tuna pâté	1.4
Vegetable pâté	2.8

JAMS AND MARMALADES	
Jam, diabetic	0.5
Jam, fruit with edible seeds	0.5
Jam, reduced sugar	0.5
Jam, stone fruit	0.5
Marmalade	0.5
Marmalade, diabetic	0.5

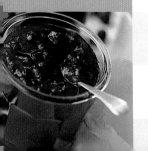

ENERGY cal	ENERGY J	FAT g	SATURATED FAT g	PROTEIN g	CARBOHYDRATE g	FIBER g
91	380	6	0.9	1	9	0.2
19	83	Trace	Trace	0	5	0.1
49	209	0	0	0	13	0
42	180	1	0.2	0	9	0
17	71	1	0.5	2	0	0
147	608	14	2.5	5	1	Trace
19	80	1	0.6	2	0	Trace
90	377	7	2.1	5	2	0.3
114	472	10	3	5	0	Trace
156	645	13	2.9	6	3	1.4
152	628	13	2.4	6	2	1.5
94	393	7	3.1	7	0	Trace
138	574	11	6	6	5	2
26	109	0	0	0	9	0.1
39	167	0	0	0	10	0.1
18	78	Trace	Trace	0	5	0.1
39	167	0	0	0	10	0.1
39	167	0	0	0	10	0
26	109	0	0	0	9	0.1

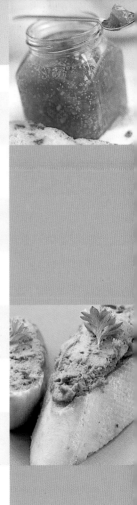

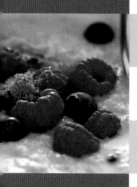

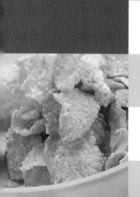

BREAKFAST CEREALS	AVERAGE PORTION oz
Bran, flakes	1
Bran, flakes with oat	1
Bran, strands	1.4
Bran, raisin	1
Bran, with oat and wheat	1.8
Corn flakes	1
Corn flakes, with nuts	1
Crunchy clusters with fruit	1.8
Frosted flakes	1
Fruit and fibre breakfast cereal	1.4
Hoops, honey	1
Hoops, honey and nut	1
Malted flakes	1
Muesli	1.8
Muesli, Swiss-style	1.8
Muesli, with extra fruit	1.8
Muesli, with no added sugar	1.8
Multigrain flakes	1
Oat cereal with fruit and nuts	1.8
Oat cereal with tropical fruit	1.8
Oat clusters	1
Oat flakes	1
Oatmeal, instant, made with water	6.3
Oatmeal, made with milk and water	5.6
Oatmeal, made with water	5.6
Oatmeal, made with whole milk	5.6
Puffed rice	1
Puffed rice, chocolate	1
Puffed wheat	0.7
Wheat, shredded	1.6
Wheat, shredded, honey and nut	1.4
Wheat, shredded, mini	1.6
Wholewheat biscuits	0.7

All values are without any sugar added.

ENERGY cal	ENERGY J	FAT g	SATURATED FAT g	PROTEIN g	CARBOHYDRATE g	FIBER g
95	406	1	0.1	3	21	3.9
105	435	2	0.2	3	20	3
104	444	1	0.2	6	19	9.8
96	405	1	0.1	3	18	3.9
163	691	2	0.3	5	34	8.9
108	461	Trace	0	2	26	0.3
119	507	1	0.2	2	27	0.2
130	680	5	1.7	4	20	1.3
113	482	Trace	0	2	28	0.2
147	614	2	1.2	2	28	2.2
111	465	1	0.2	2	23	2.1
112	474	1	0.3	2	23	1.5
186	773	1	0.1	3	23	1.3
184	770	3	0.7	6	33	3.2
182	770	3	0.4	5	36	3.2
186	789	3	0.4	5	37	3.2
183	776	4	0.8	5	34	3.8
111	465	Trace	Trace	5	22	0.7
213	888	8	3	5	31	2
217	905	7	4	4	34	3
116	490	3	0.8	3	20	2.7
107	456	1	0.2	3	22	3
671	2844	14	2.2	21	123	13
133	557	5	2.3	5	18	1.3
78	334	2	0.3	2	14	1.3
186	781	8	4.3	8	22	1.3
111	472	0.1	0.1	2	27	0.2
115	491	0.1	0.1	2	28	0.2
64	273	Trace	0	3	13	1.1
150	630	1	0.2	5	30	5.2
152	642	3	0.9	4	28	4.1
154	655	1	0.2	4	32	5
70	300	0.1	0.1	2	15	1.9

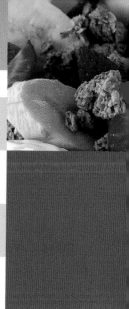

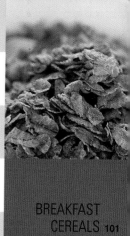

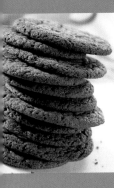

CRACKERS	**AVERAGE PORTION oz**
Cheese, low sodium	0.5
Cheese, regular	0.5
Cheese, sandwich with peanut butter	0.5
Crackers, regular	0.5
Crackers, regular, low salt	0.5
Crackers, sandwich, with cheese	0.5
Crackers, sandwich, with peanut butter	0.5
Milk crackers	0.8
Nabisco wheat thins	1
Rye, sandwich with cheese	0.5
Rye, wafers, plain	0.9
Rye, wafers, seasoned	0.8
Saltines, regular	0.5
Saltines, fat-free, low-sodium	0.5
Saltines, low salt	0.5
Saltines, unsalted tops	0.5
Wheat, low salt	0.5
Wheat, regular	0.5
Wheat, sandwich, with cheese	0.5
Wheat, sandwich, with peanut butter	0.5
Wholewheat	0.5
Wholewheat, low salt	0.5

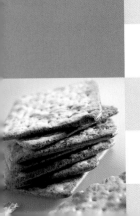

CRISPBREADS	
Breadsticks (4)	0.9
Crispbakes	0.6
Crispbread, rye	0.5
Matzo, egg	0.5
Matzo, egg and onion	0.5
Matzo, plain	0.5
Matzo, wholewheat	0.5
Melba toast, plain	0.5
Melba toast, plain, without salt	0.5

Unless otherwise specified, a helping is two biscuits.

ENERGY cal	ENERGY J	FAT g	SATURATED FAT g	PROTEIN g	CARBOHYDRATE g	FIBER g
75	316	4	1.4	2	9	0.4
75	316	4	1.4	2	9	0.4
72	303	3	0.8	2	9	0.4
75	315	4	0.6	1	9	0.2
75	315	4	0.6	1	9	0.2
72	299	3	0.9	1	9	0.3
73	306	4	0.8	2	9	0.4
100	419	3	0.6	2	15	0.4
136	570	6	0.9	2	20	0.9
67	282	3	0.8	1	9	0.5
84	349	0	0	2	20	5.7
84	351	2	0.3	2	16	4.6
65	272	2	0.4	1	11	0.4
59	247	0	0	2	12	0.4
65	272	2	0.4	1	11	0.4
65	272	2	0.4	1	11	0.4
71	297	3	0.8	1	10	0.7
71	297	3	0.8	1	10	0.7
75	312	4	0.6	1	9	0.5
74	311	4	0.7	2	8	0.7
66	278	3	0.5	1	10	1.6
66	278	3	0.5	1	10	1.6
108	464	4	1.6	4	20	0.8
60	250	Trace	Trace	2	12	0.6
55	230	0	0	1	12	2.5
59	245	0	0.1	2	12	0.4
59	245	1	0.1	2	12	0.8
59	248	0	0	2	13	0.4
53	220	0	0	2	12	1.8
58	245	0	0.1	2	11	0.9
58	245	0	0.1	2	11	0.9

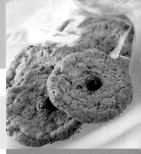

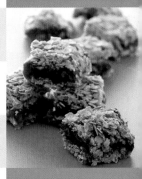

COOKIES & CRACKERS 103

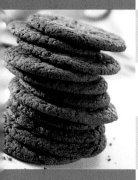

	AVERAGE PORTION oz
CRISPBREADS	
Melba toast, rye	0.5
Melba toast, wheat	0.5
Rice cakes	0.6
COOKIES	
Animal crackers	0.5
Archway, apple-filled oatmeal	0.9
Archway, coconut macaroon	0.8
Archway, date-filled oatmeal	0.9
Archway, fat-free oatmeal raisin	1.1
Archway, fat-free oatmeal raspberry	1.1
Archway, gourmet oatmeal pecan	1
Archway, gourmet Ruth's golden oatmeal	1
Archway, iced oatmeal	1
Archway, oatmeal	0.9
Archway, oatmeal raisin	0.9
Archway, Ruth's oatmeal	0.9
Archway, sugar-free oatmeal	0.8
Chocolate chip	0.8
Chocolate grahams	1
Chocolate sandwich, with creme filling, chocolate-coated	1.2
Chocolate wafers	0.5
Coconut macaroons, homemade	0.8
Fig bars	1.2
Marshmallows, chocolate-coated	0.9
Oatmeal, homemade, with raisins	1.1
Oatmeal, homemade, without raisins	1.1
Oatmeal, refrigerated dough, baked	0.8
Oatmeal, store-bought, fat-free	1
Oatmeal, store-bought, regular	0.8
Oatmeal, store-bought, soft-type	1.1
Oatmeal, store-bought, special dietary	1

Unless otherwise specified, a helping is two biscuits.

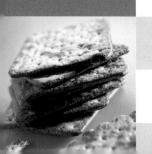

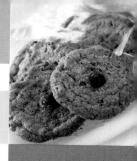

ENERGY cal	ENERGY J	FAT g	SATURATED FAT g	PROTEIN g	CARBOHYDRATE g	FIBER g
58	244	1	0.1	2	12	1.2
56	235	0	0.1	2	11	1.1
56	234	Trace	Trace	2	12	0.8
67	280	2	0.5	1	11	0.2
98	412	3	0.7	1	16	0.5
106	444	6	5.4	1	12	0.5
99	413	3	0.7	1	17	0.7
106	445	0	0.1	1	24	0.9
109	455	0	0.1	1	25	0.9
134	559	7	2.4	2	16	0.8
122	508	5	1	2	18	0.8
123	514	5	1.5	1	18	0.6
106	444	4	0.9	2	17	0.7
107	446	4	0.8	1	17	0.8
111	466	4	0.9	2	17	0.7
106	444	5	1.2	1	16	0.5
112	461	6	2.7	1	14	0.4
136	567	6	3.7	2	19	0.9
164	684	9	2.5	1	22	1.8
52	217	2	0.5	1	9	0.4
97	406	3	2.7	1	17	0.4
111	466	2	0.4	1	23	1.5
109	458	4	1.2	1	18	0.5
130	546	5	1	2	21	0.8
134	561	5	1.1	2	20	0.8
113	473	5	1.3	1	16	0.7
91	382	0	0.1	2	22	2
112	471	5	1.1	2	17	0.7
123	513	4	1.1	2	20	0.8
126	526	5	0.8	1	20	0.8

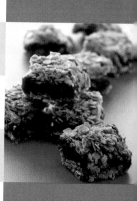

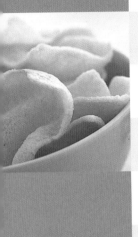

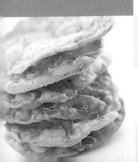

SAVORY SNACKS	AVERAGE PORTION oz
Bombay mix	1
Breadsticks	0.9
Cheese and potato puffs	0.9
Cheese balls	1.2
Chips, corn-based, plain	1
Corn snacks	0.9
Oriental mix	1.8
Popcorn, candied	2.6
Popcorn, salted	2.6
Pork scratchings	0.8
Potato and corn sticks	0.7
Potato and corn, waffle-shaped snacks	1.8
Potato crisps	1
Potato crisps, crinkle cut	1.4
Potato crisps, jacket	1.4
Potato crisps, low-fat	1
Potato crisps, square	0.8
Potato crisps, thick, crinkle cut	1.4
Potato crisps, thick cut	1.4
Potato rings	1
Pretzels	1
Taco chips	0.9
Tortilla chips, nacho-flavor	1
Tortilla chips, nacho-flavor, light	1
Tortilla chips, nacho-flavor, made with enriched masa flour	1
Tortilla chips, plain	1
Tortilla chips, ranch-flavor	1
Tortilla chips, taco-flavor	1
Trail mix	0.8

ENERGY cal	ENERGY J	FAT g	SATURATED FAT g	PROTEIN g	CARBOHYDRATE g	FIBER g
151	630	10	1.2	6	11	1.9
108	464	4	1.6	4	20	0.8
140	585	9	3.2	2	15	0.3
148	621	8	1.8	2	19	0.8
151	631	9	1.3	2	16	1.4
141	591	9	3.8	1	16	1
273	1142	20	3	10	17	0.3
360	1514	14	1.5	2	58	1
445	1851	32	3.2	5	37	1
133	554	10	3.6	11	0	0.1
88	368	4	1.3	1	11	0.6
241	1009	12	2.8	2	32	1.3
159	665	10	4.2	2	16	1.6
219	913	14	5.8	2	22	2.3
204	851	13	5.3	3	21	1.9
137	577	6	2.8	2	19	1.8
108	454	5	2.2	2	14	1.1
203	848	12	5	2	22	1.6
200	836	11	4.6	3	23	1.6
157	656	10	4.2	1	18	0.8
114	479	1	0.2	3	24	0.8
124	521	6	1.6	1	17	1.8
139	584	7	1.4	2	17	1.5
125	521	4	0.8	2	20	1.3
139	584	7	1.4	2	17	1.5
140	587	7	1.4	2	18	1.8
137	574	7	1.3	2	18	1.1
134	562	7	1.3	2	18	1.5
108	451	7	1.3	2	9	1.1

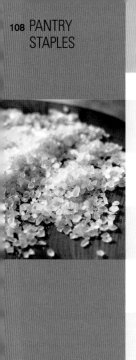

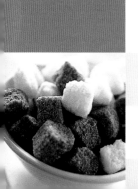

FLOUR	AVERAGE PORTION OZ
Corn starch	1
Rye, whole	0.7
Wheat, brown	3.5
Wheat, white, bread	3.5
Wheat, white, all-purpose	3.5
Wheat, white, self-rising	3.5
Wheat, wholewheat	3.5

GRAVY AND STOCK	
Fish stock, homemade	8.2
Gravy, chicken, canned	8.4
Gravy, au jus, canned	8.4
Gravy, beef, canned	8.2
Gravy, instant granules	0.2
Gravy, mushroom, canned	8.4
Gravy, turkey, canned	8.4
Stock cubes, beef/chicken	0.25
Stock cubes, vegetable	0.25

MISCELLANEOUS	
Baking soda	0.2
Bran, wheat	0.25
Coconut, creamed block	0.8
Coconut, desiccated	0.9
Gelatine	0.1
Marzipan, store bought	0.8
Olives, in brine, pitted	0.6
Pancake mix, plain (with buttermilk)	3.5
Pancake mix, wholewheat	3.5
Tomato purée	0.7
Tomatoes, sundried, bottled in oil	0.4
Vegetable purée	0.7

ENERGY cal	ENERGY J	FAT g	SATURATED FAT g	PROTEIN g	CARBOHYDRATE g	FIBER g
106	452	0	0	0	28	0
67	286	1	0.1	2	15	2.3
323	1377	2	0.2	13	69	6.4
341	1451	1	0.2	12	75	3.1
341	1450	1	0.2	9	78	3.1
330	1407	1	0.2	9	76	3.1
310	1318	2	0.3	13	64	9
40	165	2	0.5	5	0	0
188	788	14	3.4	5	13	1
38	159	0	0.2	3	6	0
123	517	5	2.7	9	11	0.9
23	96	2	Trace	0	2	Trace
119	497	6	1	3	13	1
121	507	5	1.5	6	12	1
17	69	1	Trace	1	1	0
18	74	1	Trace	1	1	Trace
0	0	0	0	0	0	0
14	61	1	0.1	1	2	2.5
167	690	17	14.8	2	2	2
169	698	17	15	2	2	3.8
10	43	0	0	3	0	0
101	426	3	0.3	1	17	0.5
19	76	2	0.3	0	Trace	0.5
376	1573	5	1	10	71	2.7
344	1439	2	0.2	13	71	2
15	65	Trace	Trace	1	3	0.6
50	204	5	0.7	0	1	0.5
14	51	1	0	1	1	0.6

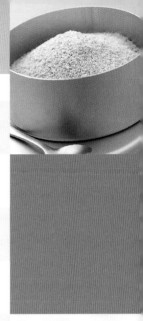

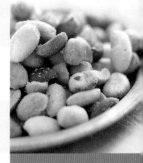

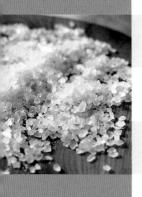

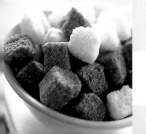

MISCELLANEOUS	AVERAGE PORTION OZ
Vinegar	0.5
Vinegar, cider	0.5
Wheatgerm	0.2
Yeast, bakers', compressed	0.2
Yeast, dried	0.2

SUGARS, SYRUPS AND TREACLE	
Sugar, brown	0.7
Sugar, Demerara	0.7
Sugar, icing	0.7
Sugar, white	0.7
Syrup, golden	1.9
Syrup, golden, pouring	1.8
Syrup, maple	1.9
Treacle, black	1.8

NUTS AND SEEDS	
Almonds, toasted	0.5
Brazil nuts	0.4
Cashew nuts, plain	0.4
Cashew nuts, roasted and salted	0.8
Chestnuts	50
Coconut, fresh	0.9
Hazelnuts	0.4
Macadamia nuts, salted	0.4
Mixed nuts	1.4
Mixed nuts and raisins	1.4
Peanuts, dry roasted	1.4
Peanuts, plain	0.5
Peanuts, roasted and salted	0.8
Pecan nuts	2
Pine nuts	0.2

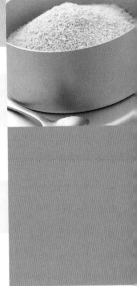

ENERGY cal	ENERGY J	FAT g	SATURATED FAT g	PROTEIN g	CARBOHYDRATE g	FIBER g
3	13	0	0	0	0	0
2	9	0	0	0	1	0
18	75	0	0.1	1	2	0.8
3	11	0	0	1	0	Trace
8	36	0	0	2	0	Trace
72	309	0	0	0	20	0
79	336	0	0	0	21	0
79	336	0	0	Trace	21	0
79	336	0	0	Trace	21	0
164	698	0	0	0	43	0
148	632	0	0	Trace	40	0
144	602	Trace	Trace	0	37	0
129	548	0	0	1	34	Trace
81	334	7	0.6	3	1	1
68	281	7	1.6	1	0	0.4
57	237	5	1	2	2	0.3
153	633	13	2.5	5	5	0.8
85	360	1	0.3	1	18	2
98	405	10	8.7	1	1	2
65	269	6	0.5	1	1	0.7
75	308	8	1.1	1	0	0.5
243	1006	22	3.4	9	3	2.4
192	802	14	2.2	6	13	1.8
236	976	20	3.6	10	4	2.6
73	304	6	1.1	3	2	0.8
151	623	13	2.4	6	2	1.5
413	1706	42	3.4	6	3	2.8
34	142	3	0.2	1	0	0.1

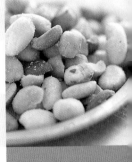

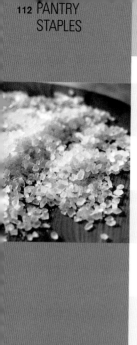

NUTS AND SEEDS

	AVERAGE PORTION OZ
Pistachio nuts, roasted and salted	0.4
Pumpkin seeds	0.6
Sesame seeds	0.5
Sunflower seeds	0.6
Walnuts	0.7

SOUP

Beef broth	8.5
Beef noodle	8.6
Black bean	8.7
Chicken broth	8.5
Chicken corn chowder, chunky	8.5
Chicken gumbo	8.6
Chicken noodle, chunky	8.6
Crab	8.6
Gazpacho	8.6
Mushroom barley	8.6
Tomato rice	8.7
Tomato	8.7
Turkey noodle	8.6
Vegetable	8.5

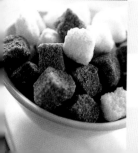

All soups are canned.

ENERGY cal	ENERGY J	FAT g	SATURATED FAT g	PROTEIN g	CARBOHYDRATE g	FIBER g
60	249	6	0.7	2	1	0.6
91	378	7	1.1	4	2	0.8
72	296	7	1	2	0	0.9
96	400	8	0.8	3	3	1
138	567	14	1.1	3	1	0.7
17	70	1	0.3	3	0	0
83	346	3	1.1	5	9	0.7
116	487	2	0.4	6	20	4.4
38	161	1	0.4	5	1	0
238	994	15	4.2	7	18	2.2
56	234	1	0.3	3	8	2
114	479	3	0.8	8	14	2
76	317	2	0.4	5	10	0.7
46	193	0	0	7	4	0.5
73	307	2	0.4	2	12	0.7
119	496	3	0.5	2	22	1.5
161	675	6	2.9	6	22	2.7
68	285	2	0.6	4	9	0.7
72	304	2	0.3	2	12	0.5

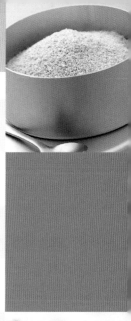

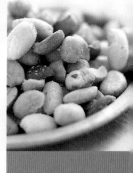

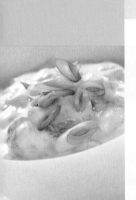

TABLE SAUCES	AVERAGE PORTION oz
Applesauce, homemade	0.7
Applesauce, sweetened, canned	1
Applesauce, unsweetened, canned	1.3
Chili sauce	0.8
Cranberry sauce, canned, sweetened	2
Horseradish sauce	0.7
Mint sauce	0.4
Mustard, powder, made up	0.3
Mustard, smooth	0.1
Mustard, wholegrain	0.5
Soy sauce, dark, thick	0.2
Soy sauce, light, thin	0.2
Tartar sauce	1
Tomato ketchup	0.7

DRESSINGS AND MAYONNAISE

Blue and roquefort cheese dressing	0.5
Blue cheese dressing	0.8
'Fat-free' dressing	0.5
French dressing	0.5
French dressing, diet, low fat	0.6
Italian dressing, diet	0.5
Italian dressing	0.5
Kraft Free fat free Italian dressing	0.5
Kraft Free fat free ranch dressing	0.5
Kraft Free fat free ranch dressing	0.5
Kraft Light Done Right! Italian dressing	0.5
Kraft Light Done Right! ranch dressing	0.5
Kraft fat free mayonnaise dressing	0.6
Kraft light mayonnaise	0.5
Kraft Miracle Whip Free nonfat dressing	0.6
Kraft Miracle Whip Light dressing	0.6
Kraft ranch dressing	0.5

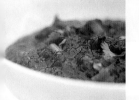

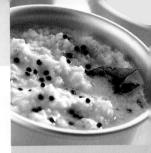

ENERGY cal	ENERGY J	FAT g	SATURATED FAT g	PROTEIN g	CARBOHYDRATE g	FIBER g
13	55	0	0	0	3	0.2
23	95	0	0	0	6	0.4
15	63	0	0	0	4	0.4
20	84	Trace	Trace	0	4	0.3
86	360	0	0	0	22	0.6
31	128	2	0.2	1	4	0.5
10	43	Trace	Trace	0	2	0.2
18	75	1	0.1	1	0	0
3	12	0	0	0	0	0
20	82	1	0.1	1	5	Trace
3	13	0	0	0	6	0.2
3	13	Trace	Trace	0	1	0.7
90	372	7	0.5	0	0	0.2
23	98	Trace	Trace	0	1	0.7
76	316	8	1.5	1	1	0
114	472	12	6.2	1	2	0
10	42	0	0	0	2	0
64	270	6	1.4	0	3	0
21	90	1	0.1	0	3	0
16	66	1	0.2	0	1	0
70	293	7	1	0	2	0
9	39	0	0.1	0	2	0.1
21	87	0	0	0	5	0.1
21	87	0	0	0	5	0.1
26	107	2	0.2	0	1	0.2
38	161	3	0.3	0	2	0.1
11	47	0	0.1	0	2	0.3
50	210	5	0.8	0	1	0
13	56	0	0.1	0	2	0.3
37	155	3	0.5	0	2	0
76	320	8	1.2	0	1	0

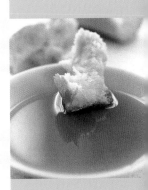

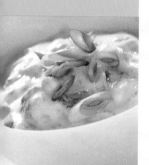

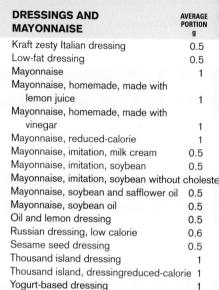

DRESSINGS AND MAYONNAISE	AVERAGE PORTION g
Kraft zesty Italian dressing	0.5
Low-fat dressing	0.5
Mayonnaise	1
Mayonnaise, homemade, made with lemon juice	1
Mayonnaise, homemade, made with vinegar	1
Mayonnaise, reduced-calorie	1
Mayonnaise, imitation, milk cream	0.5
Mayonnaise, imitation, soybean	0.5
Mayonnaise, imitation, soybean without choleste	
Mayonnaise, soybean and safflower oil	0.5
Mayonnaise, soybean oil	0.5
Oil and lemon dressing	0.5
Russian dressing, low calorie	0.6
Sesame seed dressing	0.5
Thousand island dressing	1
Thousand island, dressingreduced-calorie	1
Yogurt-based dressing	1

WHITE SAUCES	
Cheese sauce, made with low-fat milk	2.2
Cheese sauce, made with whole milk	2.2
Onion sauce, made with low-fat milk	2.2
Onion sauce, made with whole milk	2.2
White sauce, savory, made with low-fat milk	2.2
White sauce, savory, made with whole milk	2.2
White sauce, sweet, made with low-fat milk	2.2
White sauce, sweet, made with whole milk	2.2

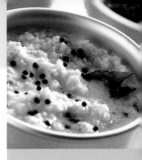

ENERGY kcal	ENERGY kJ	FAT g	SATURATED FAT g	PROTEIN g	CARBOHYDRATE g	FIBRE g
53	220	5	0.6	0	1	0.1
11	45	1	0.1	0	1	Trace
207	853	23	3.3	0	1	0
237	974	26	3.8	1	0	Trace
217	894	24	3.5	1	0	0
86	356	0	1.1	0	2	0
14	61	1	0.4	0	2	0
35	145	3	0.5	0	2	0
0.5	67	282	7	1	0	2 0
100	420	11	1.2	0	0	0
100	420	11	1.7	0	0	0
97	399	11	1.1	0	0	Trace
23	95	1	0.1	0	4	0
66	278	7	0.9	0	1	0.2
97	401	9	0.9	0	4	0.1
59	243	5	0.5	0	4	Trace
88	363	8	0.8	1	3	Trace
112	465	8	3.9	4	6	0.1
122	508	8	4.8	4	6	0.1
53	224	3	1.1	2	5	0.2
61	257	4	1.7	2	5	0.2
79	334	5	1.8	3	7	0.1
93	387	6	2.7	3	7	0.1
93	393	4	1.7	2	12	0.1
105	441	6	2.5	2	12	0.1

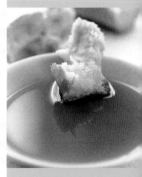

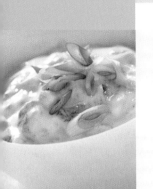

CHUTNEYS

	AVERAGE PORTION g
Chutney, apple, homemade	1.2
Chutney, mango, oily	1.2
Chutney, mango, sweet	1.2
Chutney, mixed fruit	1.2
Chutney, tomato	1.2

DIPS

Dips, sour-cream-based	1
Guacamole	1.6
Hummus	1
Taramasalata	1.6
Tzatziki	1.6

PICKLES

Gherkins, pickled	0.8
Onions, pickled	1
Pickle, chilli, oily	0.5
Pickle, lime, oily	0.5
Pickle, mango, oily	0.5
Pickle, mixed vegetables	0.5
Pickle, sweet	0.5

COOKING SAUCES

Barbecue sauce	0.8
Black bean sauce	0.7
Chili sauce	0.8
Cook-in-sauces, canned, different flavors	5.3
Curry sauce, canned	5.3
Curry sauce, sweet	5.3
Curry sauce with tomato and onion	5.3

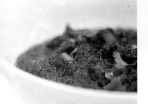

ENERGY kcal	ENERGY kJ	FAT g	SATURATED FAT g	PROTEIN g	CARBOHYDRATE g	FIBRE g
66	283	Trace	Trace	0	17	0.4
94	397	4	Trace	0	16	0.3
62	266	Trace	Trace	0	16	0.3
51	219	Trace	Traoo	0	13	0.3
42	179	Trace	Trace	0	10	0.4
108	445	11	3.7	1	1	Trace
58	239	6	1.2	1	1	1.1
56	234	4	0.5	2	3	0.7
227	935	24	1.8	1	2	Trace
30	124	2	1.3	2	1	0.1
4	15	Trace	Trace	0	1	0.3
7	30	Trace	Trace	0	1	0.4
41	168	4	Trace	0	1	0.2
27	111	2	Trace	0	1	0.2
27	110	2	Trace	0	1	0.2
3	14	0	0	0	1	0.2
21	91	0	Trace	0	5	0.2
23	99	0	0	0	6	0.1
19	79	0	0	1	2	0.4
20	84	Trace	Trace	0	4	0.3
65	272	4	0.2	2	12	Trace
117	486	8	0.4	2	11	Trace
137	570	8	2.3	2	14	2.1
297	1229	29	3	3	9	1.7

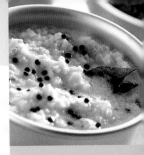

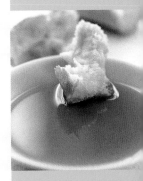

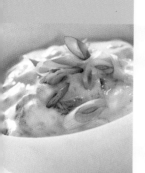

COOKING SAUCES

	AVERAGE PORTION g
Fish sauce	0.7
Hoisin sauce	0.6
Nestlé, Contadina Spaghetti Sauce, ready-to-serve	4.4
Oyster sauce	0.5
Pasta sauce, tomato based	6
Plum sauce	0.7
Prego Traditional 100% Natural Spaghetti Sauce, jar	4.6
Sofrito sauce	0.5
Soy sauce, dark, thick	0.2
Soy sauce, light, thin	0.2
Spaghetti marinara sauce, ready-to-serve	4.4
Spaghetti sauce, meatless, canned	9.6
Tabasco	0.2
Teriyaki sauce	0.7
Tomato sauce	3.2

CUSTARDS

Crème caramel	3.2
Crème patissière	5.3
Custard, made with low-fat milk	5.3
Custard, made with whole milk	4.2

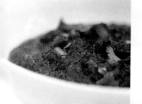

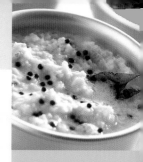

ENERGY kcal	ENERGY kJ	FAT g	SATURATED FAT g	PROTEIN g	CARBOHYDRATE g	FIBRE g
6	26	0	0	1	1	0
35	147	1	0.1	1	7	0.4
70	292	2	0.2	2	12	2.4
12	51	0	Trace	1	3	Trace
80	340	3	0.3	3	12	2.5
35	146	0	0	0	8	0.1
136	569	5	1.1	2	21	4
36	149	3	0	2	1	0.3
3	13	0	0	0	0	00
3	13	0	0	0	0	0
71	298	3	0.4	2	10	2
129	541	2	0.4	3	23	3
1	2	0	0	0	0	0
15	63	0	0	1	3	0
80	337	5	1.6	2	8	1.3
98	416	1	Trace	3	19	Trace
255	1077	9	4.1	10	37	0.3
141	605	3	1.8	6	25	Trace
140	594	5	3.4	4	20	Trace

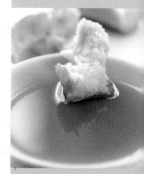

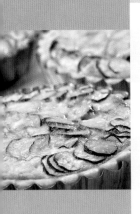

PASTRY	AVERAGE PORTION oz
Cheese	3.5
Choux	3.5
Flaky	3.5
Pie	3.5
Puff	1.4
Wholewheat	3.5

SWEET PASTRIES

Asian pastries	1.4
Chinese flaky pastries	1.4
Croissants, plain	2
Danish pastry, cheese	2.5
Danish pastry, cinnamon	1.9
Danish pastry, fruit	1.9
Danish pastry, nut	1.9
Danish pastry, raspberry	2.5
Greek pastries	3.5

PASTRY DISHES

Beef pie, shop bought	5
Chicken and mushroom pie	3.5
Chicken pie, individual, baked	4.6
Quiche, broccoli	5
Quiche, broccoli, wholewheat	5
Quiche, cauliflower and cheese	5
Quiche, cauliflower and cheese, wholewheat	5
Quiche, cheese and egg	5
Quiche, cheese and egg, wholewheat	5
Quiche, cheese and mushroom	5
Quiche, cheese and mushroom, wholewheat	5

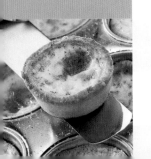

ENERGY cal	ENERGY J	FAT g	SATURATED FAT g	PROTEIN g	CARBOHYDRATE g	FIBER g
500	2083	34	15.3	13	37	1.5
325	1355	20	15	9	30	1.2
560	2332	41	14.7	6	46	1.8
521	2174	32	11.7	7	54	2.2
223	934	15	2.2	3	18	0.6
499	2080	33	11.8	9	45	6.3
215	897	16	8	3	17	0.8
157	659	7	4	2	24	0.8
224	938	12	5.9	5	26	1.0
266	1111	16	4.8	6	26	0.7
214	894	12	3	4	24	0.7
197	823	10	2.6	3	25	1
228	953	13	3.1	4	24	1.1
263	1102	13	2	4	34	1.3
322	1349	17	9	5	40	0.8
437	1826	24	11.8	12	38	0.7
200	836	10	4.5	13	14	0.6
374	1563	21	9.1	12	32	1
349	1455	21	8.3	12	30	1.7
337	1408	21	8.3	13	25	3.8
277	1156	18	7.1	7	24	1.5
269	1121	18	7.1	8	20	3.1
440	1834	31	14.4	18	24	0.8
431	1796	31	14.6	18	20	2.7
396	1655	26	10.8	15	26	1.3
388	1616	27	10.8	16	22	3.1

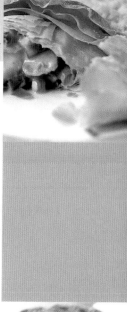

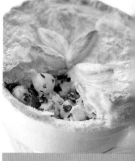

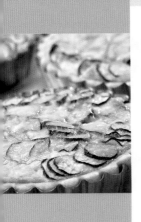

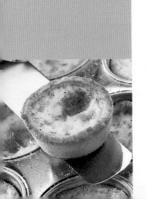

TOASTER PASTRIES	AVERAGE PORTION g
Quiche, cheese, onion and potato	5
Quiche, cheese, onion and potato, wholewheat	5
Quiche, mushroom	5
Quiche, mushroom, wholewheat	5
Quiche, spinach	5
Quiche, spinach, wholewheat	5
Quiche, vegetable	5
Quiche, vegetable, wholewheat	5
Kellogg's Pop-Tarts, apple cinnamon	1.8
Kellogg's Pop-Tarts, blueberry	1.8
Kellogg's Pop-Tarts, brown sugar cinnamon	1.8
Kellogg's Pop-Tarts, cherry	1.8
Kellogg's Pop-Tarts, frosted blueberry	1.8
Kellogg's Pop-Tarts, frosted brown sugar cinnamon	1.8
Kellogg's Pop-Tarts, frosted cherry	1.8
Kellogg's Pop-Tarts, frosted chocolate fudge	1.8
Kellogg's Pop-Tarts, frosted chocolate vanilla creme	1.8
Kellogg's Pop-Tarts, frosted grape	1.8
Kellogg's Pop-Tarts, frosted raspberry	1.8
Kellogg's Pop-Tarts, frosted strawberry	1.8
Kellogg's Pop-Tarts, frosted wild berry	1.9
Kellogg's Pop-Tarts, milk chocolate	1.8
Kellogg's Pop-Tarts, strawberry	1.8
Kellogg's Pop-Tarts Pastry Swirls, apple cinnamon Danish	2.1
Kellogg's Pop-Tarts Pastry Swirls, cheese Danish	2.1
Kellogg's Pop-Tarts Pastry Swirls, strawberry Danish	2.1

ENERGY kcal	ENERGY kJ	FAT g	SATURATED FAT g	PROTEIN g	CARBOHYDRATE g	FIBRE g
480	2005	33	16	18	28	1.4
472	1966	34	16.1	19	25	3.1
398	1659	27	12.2	14	26	1.3
388	1618	28	12.2	15	21	3.1
287	1203	18	5.6	14	18	2
281	1176	18	5.6	15	16	3.2
295	1230	18	6	7	28	2.1
286	1197	18	6	8	24	3.9
205	860	5	0.9	2	37	0.6
212	888	7	1.1	2	36	0.6
219	916	9	1	3	32	0.8
204	855	5	0.9	2	37	0.6
203	851	5	1	2	37	0.6
211	883	7	1.1	2	34	0.6
204	855	5	1	2	37	0.5
201	842	5	1	3	37	0.6
203	851	5	1	3	37	0.5
203	851	5	0.9	2	38	0.5
205	860	6	1	2	37	0.5
203	849	5	1.4	2	38	0.5
210	876	5	1.4	2	39	0.5
205	860	6	1.5	3	36	0.8
205	857	5	1.5	2	37	0.6
256	1071	11	3	3	37	0.9
252	1056	11	3	3	37	0.3
254	1063	11	3	3	37	1.1

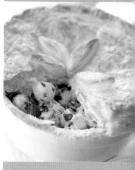

PASTRY &
PASTRY DISHES 125

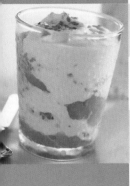

MILK-BASED PUDDINGS AND DESSERTS	AVERAGE PORTION OZ
Milk pudding, made with low-fat milk	7
Milk pudding, made with whole milk	7
Rice desserts, individual, with fruit	4.8
Rice pudding, canned	7
Tiramisu	3.2
Trifle, chocolate	4
Trifle, fruit	4

CHEESECAKES

Chocolate	4.2
Frozen	3.2
Fruit, individual	3.2
Fruit, large	4.2

OTHER DESSERTS

Crumble, fruit	6
Jelly, made with water	4
Plum pudding	3.5
Profiteroles with chocolate sauce	5.5
Strudel, fruit	4

MOUSSE

Chocolate, individual	2
Chocolate	2
Fruit	2

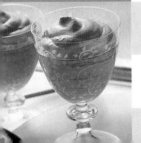

ENERGY cal	ENERGY J	FAT g	SATURATED FAT g	PROTEIN g	CARBOHYDRATE g	FIBER g
214	914	4	2.2	8	40	0.2
258	1086	9	5.4	8	40	0.2
153	648	3	2.0	4	29	0.4
178	748	3	3.2	7	28	0.4
220	919	13	7.7	4	24	0.4
233	971	17	10.7	5	15	1.4
161	672	10	6.3	3	15	2.4
415	1731	28	14.4	6	37	0.8
218	915	10	5	5	30	0.8
238	1000	11	6.8	5	31	0.9
353	1477	19	11.8	5	42	1.0
373	1571	14	6.7	4	61	2.2
70	299	0	0	1	17	0
291	1227	10	4.5	5	50	1.3
535	2226	40	21.7	9	38	1.1
279	1167	16	6.0	3	33	1.2
83	352	4	2.7	2	12	0.1
73	310	2	1.5	3	11	0.1
82	345	3	2	3	11	0.1

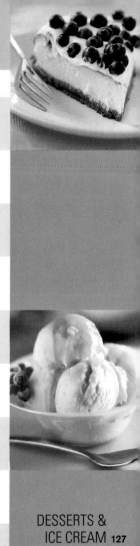

DESSERTS &

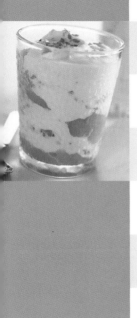

	AVERAGE PORTION oz
PIES	
Apple pie, deep filled, double crust	3.8
Apple pie, double crust	3.8
Lemon meringue pie	5.3
Mississippi mud pie	5.3
ICE CREAM AND FROZEN DESSERTS	
Banana split	3.5
Chocolate-covered ice cream bar	1.8
Chocolate nut sundae	2
Frozen ice cream dessert, chocolate	2
Frozen ice cream dessert, plain	2
Ice cream, chocolate	2.6
Ice cream, dairy-free	2.6
Ice cream, fruit	2.6
Ice cream, luxury, vanilla	2.6
Ice cream, soya	2.6
Ice cream, vanilla	2.6
Ice cream, virtually fat free	2.6
Ice cream bar, chocolate flavoured coating	1.7
Ice cream cone, chocolate/mint/nuts	2.6
Ice cream cone, strawberry	2.9
Popsicle, fruit	2.6
Creamsicle, with fruit coating	2.6
Peach melba	2
Sorbet, fruit	2.6

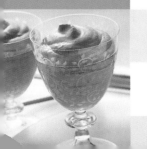

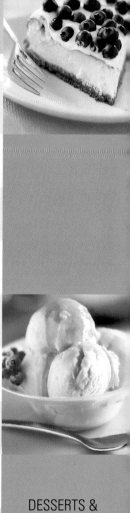

ENERGY cal	ENERGY J	FAT g	SATURATED FAT g	PROTEIN g	CARBOHYDRATE g	FIBER g
281	1183	12	3.8	4	42	1.1
269	1129	14	4.5	4	33	1.1
377	1590	13	4.6	4	65	0.7
478	1997	30	15.0	6	49	3.8
182	761	11	6	2	19	0.6
163	679	2	7.7	3	12	0
167	699	9	5	2	21	0.1
150	627	11	8.5	2	13	0.0
136	568	9	6.7	2	14	Trace
156	653	8	5.2	3	19	0.0
156	654	9	2.8	2	17	0.1
119	499	5	3.4	2	17	0.2
161	670	11	6.8	3	13	0.0
156	654	9	2.8	2	17	0.1
115	480	6	3.6	2	14	0.0
76	324	1	Trace	3	15	0.0
142	590	10	8.8	2	11	0.0
207	867	13	9.6	3	21	0.2
201	844	10	7.1	3	28	0.2
56	234	1	0.1	0	14	0.1
78	326	2	1	1	15	0.1
98	411	6	3.8	1	10	0.2
98	422	Trace	Trace	1	26	0

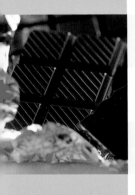

CANDY	AVERAGE PORTION OZ
Hard candy	0.25
Coconut/chocolate bar	2
Chewy candy	0.1
Chocolate, baking	1.8
Chocolate, diabetic	1.8
Chocolate, fancy and filled	8
Chocolate, milk	54
Chocolate, semisweet	1.8
Chocolate, white	1.8
Chocolate-covered bar with fruit/nut	1.2
Chocolate-covered bar with wafer/cookie	1.2
Chocolate-covered cookie fingers	0.9
Chocolate-covered caramels	0.2
Chocolate-covered wafer cookies	0.8
Creme eggs®	1.4
Fruit gums/jellies	0.1
Fudge	0.4
M&Ms®-type sweets	0.5
Marshmallows	0.2
Nougat	2.5
Peanut brittle	2
Peppermints	0.2
Toffees, mixed	0.3
Truffles, mocha	0.25
Truffles, rum	0.25

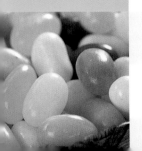

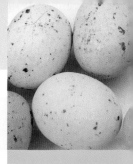

ENERGY cal	ENERGY J	FAT g	SATURATED FAT g	PROTEIN g	CARBOHYDRATE g	FIBER g
23	98	Trace	0	Trace	6	0
270	1129	15	12.1	3	33	1.4
11	48	1	0.1	0	3	0
275	1147	17	14	2	29	0.6
224	934	15	9.1	5	19	0.6
36	150	2	0.9	0	5	0.1
281	1176	17	9.9	4	31	0.4
255	1069	14	8.4	3	32	1.3
265	1106	15	9.2	4	29	0
170	711	9	4.6	3	20	1.3
170	711	9	4.6	3	20	1.3
134	564	7	3.4	2	18	0.3
23	98	1	0.5	0	3	0
110	462	6	3.8	2	14	0.2
163	681	6	1.8	2	28	0.5
6	28	0	0	0	2	Trace
49	205	2	1	0	9	0
68	288	3	1.6	1	11	0.2
16	70	0	0	0	4	0
269	1138	6	0.8	3	54	0.6
280	1178	11	3.1	5	43	1.2
24	101	0	0	0	6	0
34	143	1	0.8	0	5	0
34	143	2	1.1	0	4	0.1
36	152	2	1.4	0	3	0.1

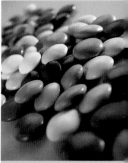

	AVERAGE PORTION fl oz
COLD BEVERAGES	
CARBONATED DRINKS	
Cola	5.6
Cola, diet	5.6
Ginger ale, dry	5.6
Ginger ale, dry, diet	5.6
Lemonade	5.6
Lemonade, diet	5.6
Orangeade	5.6
Orangeade, diet	5.6
Root beer	5.6
Soda, cream	5.6
Tonic water	5.6
FRUIT JUICES	
Apple, unsweetened	5.6
Carrot	5.6
Grape, unsweetened	5.6
Grapefruit, unsweetened	5.6
Lemon, fresh	0.4
Lime, fresh	0.4
Mango, canned	5.6
Orange, freshly squeezed	5.6
Orange, unsweetened	5.6
Passion fruit	5.6
Pineapple, unsweetened	5.6
Pomegranate, fresh	5.6
Prune	5.6
Tomato	5.6

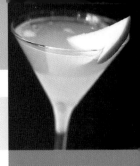

ENERGY cal	ENERGY J	FAT g	SATURATED FAT g	PROTEIN g	CARBOHYDRATE g	FIBER g
66	278	0	0	Trace	17	0
Trace	Trace	0	0	0	0	0
24	99	0	0	0	6	0
2	6	0	0	0	0.4	0
35	149	0	0	Trace	9	0
Trace	Trace	0	0	0	0	0
113	474	0	0	0	27	0
1	4	0	0	0	0.4	0
66	275	0	0	0	17	0
82	344	0	0	0	21	0
53	226	0	0	0	14	0
61	262	Trace	Trace	0	16	Trace
38	165	Trace	Trace	1	9	0.2
74	314	Trace	Trace	0	19	0
53	224	Trace	Trace	1	13	Trace
1	3	Trace	Trace	0	0	0
1	4	Trace	Trace	0	0	0
62	266	Trace	Trace	0	16	Trace
53	224	Trace	Trace	1	13	0.2
58	245	Trace	Trace	1	14	0.2
75	302	Trace	Trace	1	17	Trace
66	283	Trace	Trace	0	17	Trace
70	302	Trace	Trace	0	19	Trace
91	389	Trace	Trace	1	23	Trace
22	99	Trace	Trace	1	5	1

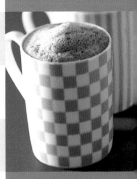

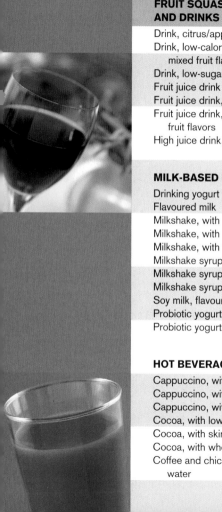

FRUIT SQUASHES AND DRINKS

	AVERAGE PORTION fl oz
Drink, citrus/apple/mixed fruit flavours	8.8
Drink, low-calorie, lemon/orange/ mixed fruit flavors	8.8
Drink, low-sugar, fortified with vitamins	8.8
Fruit juice drink	7.3
Fruit juice drink, carbonated	5.6
Fruit juice drink, low calorie, mixed fruit flavors	7.3
High juice drink, orange/lemon flavors	8.8

MILK-BASED DRINKS

Drinking yogurt	7
Flavoured milk	7.5
Milkshake, with low-fat milk	10.5
Milkshake, with skim milk	10.5
Milkshake, with whole milk	10.5
Milkshake syrup, with low-fat milk	10.2
Milkshake syrup, with skim milk	10.2
Milkshake syrup, with whole milk	10.4
Soy milk, flavoured	5.2
Probiotic yogurt drink, orange	3.5
Probiotic yogurt drink, plain	3.5

HOT BEVERAGES

Cappuccino, with low-fat milk	10.2
Cappuccino, with skim milk	10.2
Cappuccino, with whole milk	10.2
Cocoa, with low-fat milk	8.8
Cocoa, with skim milk	8.8
Cocoa, with whole milk	8.8
Coffee and chicory essence, with water	10.2

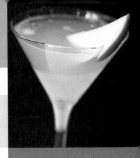

ENERGY cal	ENERGY J	FAT g	SATURATED FAT g	PROTEIN g	CARBOHYDRATE g	FIBER g
48	200	0	0	Trace	13	0
3	8	0	0	Trace	1	0
10	43	0	0	Trace	3	0
76	328	Trace	Trace	0	20	Trace
62	264	Trace	Trace	Trace	16	Trace
21	89	Trace	Trace	0	5	Trace
63	268	0	0	0	16	0
124	526	Trace	Trace	6	26	Trace
146	614	3	1.9	8	23	0
207	882	5	3	10	34	Trace
171	726	1	0.3	10	34	0
261	1104	11	7.2	9	33	Trace
171	725	4	2.6	8	27	0
136	576	1	0.2	9	27	0
223	936	10	6.2	8	27	0
58	245	2	0.3	4	5	Trace
67	279	0.9	0.6	1.5	13.4	1.3
68	284	1	0.7	1.7	13.1	1.4
46	193	2	1	3	5	0
33	141	0	0.1	3	5	0
65	269	4	2.3	3	5	0
143	608	5	3	9	18	0.5
110	475	1	0.8	9	18	0.5
190	800	10	6.5	9	17	0.5
17	76	Trace	0	0	5	0

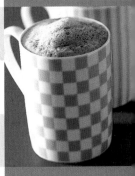

HOT DRINKS	AVERAGE PORTION fl oz
Coffee, drip	10.2
Coffee, drip, with low-fat milk	10.2
Coffee, drip, with skim milk	10.2
Coffee, drip, with single cream	10.2
Coffee, drip, with whole milk	10.2
Coffee, instant	10.2
Coffee, instant, with low-fat milk	10.2
Coffee, instant, with skim milk	10.2
Coffee, instant, with whole milk	10.2
Coffee, Irish	4.4
Drinking chocolate, with low-fat milk	10.2
Drinking chocolate, with skim milk	10.2
Drinking chocolate, with whole milk	10.2
Latte, with low-fat milk	10.2
Latte, with skim milk	10.2
Latte, with whole milk	10.2
Mocha with low-fat milk	10.2
Mocha with skim milk	10.2
Mocha with whole milk	10.2
Ovaltine, with low-fat milk	10.2
Ovaltine, with skim milk	10.2
Ovaltine, with whole milk	10.2
Tea, black	10.2
Tea, Chinese	10.2
Tea, green	10.2
Tea, herbal	10.2
Tea, lemon, instant	10.2
Tea, with low-fat milk	10.2
Tea with skim milk	10.2
Tea with whole milk	10.2

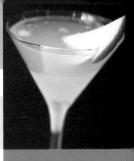

ENERGY cal	ENERGY J	FAT g	SATURATED FAT g	PROTEIN g	CARBOHYDRATE g	FIBER g
4	15	Trace	Trace	0	1	0
13	55	1	0.2	1	1	0
11	43	0	0	1	1	0
27	106	2	1.3	1	1	0
13	59	1	0.6	1	1	0
Trace	4	Trace	0	0	Trace	0
13	55	1	0.2	1	1	0
8	39	0	0	1	1	0
15	65	1	0.6	1	1	0
105	433	10	6.1	1	4	0
135	578	4	2.3	7	21	Trace
112	481	1	0.6	7	21	Trace
171	716	8	4.8	6	20	Trace
60	252	2	1.3	4	7	0
33	141	1	0.1	3	5	0
85	353	5	3	4	6	0
96	405	5	3.1	4	9	0.1
81	339	3	2	4	9	0.1
120	500	7	4.8	4	9	0.1
150	642	3	1.9	7	25	Trace
129	549	1	0.2	7	25	Trace
184	779	7	4.6	7	25	Trace
Trace	4	Trace	Trace	0	Trace	0
2	10	0	0	0	0	0
Trace	Trace	0	0	0	Trace	0
2	25	Trace	Trace	0	0	0
15	65	0	0	0	4	0
13	53	1	0.2	1	1	0
8	36	0	0	1	1	0
15	61	1	0.6	1	1	0

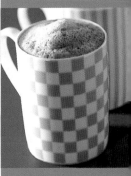

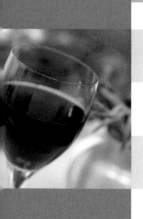

BEERS	AVERAGE PORTION fl oz
Bitter, best/premium	10
Bitter, bottled	10
Bitter, canned	10
Bitter, draft	10
Bitter, keg	10
Bitter, low-alcohol	8.8
Brown ale, bottled	8.8
Mild, draft	10
Pale ale, bottled	8.8

HARD CIDERS	
Dry	10
Low-alcohol	8.8
Sweet	10
Vintage	10

LAGERS	
Bottled	8.8
Canned	10
Draft	10
Low-alcohol	8.8
Premium	10

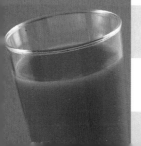

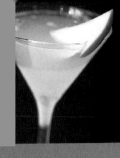

ENERGY cal	ENERGY J	FAT g	SATURATED FAT g	PROTEIN g	CARBOHYDRATE g	FIBER g
95	399	Trace	Trace	1	6	Trace
86	356	Trace	Trace	1	6	Trace
92	379	Trace	Trace	1	7	0
92	379	Trace	Trace	1	7	0
89	370	Trace	Trace	1	7	0
33	135	0	0	1	5	Trace
75	315	Trace	Trace	1	8	Trace
69	293	Trace	Trace	1	5	Trace
70	295	Trace	Trace	1	5	Trace
103	436	0	0	Trace	7	0
43	185	0	0	Trace	9	0
121	505	0	0	Trace	12	0
290	1208	0	0	Trace	21	0
73	300	Trace	Trace	1	4	0
83	347	Trace	Trace	1	Trace	Trace
83	347	Trace	Trace	1	Trace	Trace
25	103	Trace	Trace	1	4	Trace
169	700	Trace	Trace	1	7	Trace

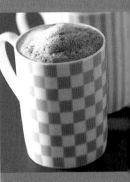

LIQUEURS	AVERAGE PORTION fl oz
Advocaat	0.9
Cherry Brandy	0.9
Cointreau	0.9
Cream liqueurs	0.9
Crème de Menthe	0.9
Curaçao	0.9
Drambuie	0.9
Egg nog	5.6
Grand Marnier	0.9
Pernod	0.9
Southern Comfort	0.9
Tia Maria	0.9

FORTIFIED WINES	
Port	1.8
Sherry, dry	1.8
Sherry, medium	1.8
Sherry, sweet	1.8
Vermouth, dry	1.7
Vermouth, sweet	1.7

SPIRITS, 40% VOLUME	
Brandy	0.9
Gin	0.9
Rum	0.9
Vodka	0.9
Whisky	0.9

ENERGY cal	ENERGY J	FAT g	SATURATED FAT g	PROTEIN g	CARBOHYDRATE g	FIBER g
65	273	2	0.5	1	7	0
66	275	0	0	Trace	8	0
79	328	0	0	Trace	6	0
81	338	4	0	Trace	6	0
66	275	0	0	Trace	8	0
78	326	0	0	Trace	7	0
79	328	0	0	Trace	6	0
102	763	7	3.4	8	18	0
79	328	0	0	Trace	6	0
79	328	0	0	Trace	6	0
79	328	0	0	Trace	6	0
66	275	0	0	Trace	8	0
79	328	0	0	0	6	0
58	241	0	0	0	1	0
58	241	0	0	0	3	0
68	284	0	0	0	3	0
52	217	0	0	0	1	0
72	303	0	0	Trace	8	0
52	215	0	0	Trace	Trace	0
52	215	0	0	Trace	Trace	0
52	215	0	0	Trace	Trace	0
52	215	0	0	Trace	Trace	0
52	215	0	0	Trace	Trace	0

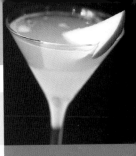

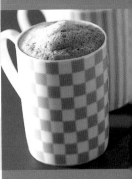

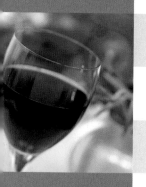

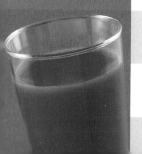

STOUT BEER	AVERAGE PORTION fl oz
Bottled	8.8
Extra	10
Guinness™	10
Mackeson	10

WINES	
Champagne	4.4
Mulled wine	4.4
Red wine	4.4
Rosé, medium	4.4
White wine, dry	4.4
White wine, medium	4.4
White wine, sparkling	4.4
White wine, sweet	4.4

COCKTAILS	
Daiquiri, canned	1
Pina colada	1.1
Tequila sunrise	1.1
Whiskey sour	1

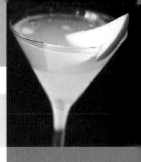

ENERGY cal	ENERGY J	FAT g	SATURATED FAT g	PROTEIN g	CARBOHYDRATE g	FIBER g
93	390	Trace	Trace	1	10	0
112	468	Trace	Trace	1	6	0
86	362	Trace	Trace	1	4	0
103	439	Trace	Trace	1	13	0
95	394	0	0	0	2	0
245	1028	0	0	0	32	0
85	354	0	0	0	0	0
89	368	0	0	0	3	0
83	344	0	0	0	1	0
93	385	0	0	0	4	0
93	384	0	0	0	6	0
118	493	0	0	0	7	0
38	157	0	0	0	5	0
76	317	2	2.1	0	9	0
35	147	0	0	0	4	0
36	149	0	0	0	4	0

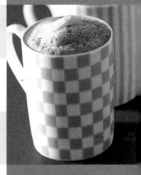

© **Burger King** 66–67.
Octopus Publishing Group Limited 123 top right, /Jean Cazals 71 bottom right, 132 top left, /Stephen Conroy 101 top right, 127 bottom right, 130 bottom left, 131 top right, /Gus Filgate 52 bottom left, /Jeremy Hopley 8 top left, 59 bottom right, 132 bottom left, /David Jordan 8 bottom left, 16 top left, 58 bottom left, 76 bottom left, 77 top right, 87 top right, 102 bottom left, 131 bottom right, 133 bottom right, /Graham Kirk 126 bottom left, /Sandra Lane 86 bottom left, 114 bottom left, /William Lingwood 16 bottom left, 17 top right, 17 bottom right, 71 top right, 76 top left, 77 bottom right, 99 bottom right, 103 bottom right, 109 top right, /Neil Mersh 58 top left, 59 top left, /Peter Myers 52 top left, 130 top left, /Sean Myers 70 top left, 70 bottom left, /William Reavell 34 top left, 34 bottom left, 35 top right, 53 top right, 53 bottom right, 80 bottom left, 94 top left, 95 top right, 98 top left, 100 top left, 100 bottom left, 101 bottom right, 106 top left, 106 bottom left, 107 bottom right, 108 top left, 108 bottom left, 114 top left, 115 top right, 126 top left, 127 top right, 133 top right, /Simon Smith 80 top left, 81 top right, 81 bottom right, 95 bottom right, 102 top left, 103 top right, 107 top right, 122 top left, 122 bottom left, /Ian Wallace 9 top right, 9 bottom right, 86 top left, 87 bottom right, 94 bottom left, 99 top right, 109 bottom right, 115 bottom right, /Philip Webb 35 bottom right, 98 bottom left, 123 bottom right.
© **Kentucky Fried Chicken** 68–69.

Commissioning Editor Nicola Hill
Editorial Director Jane Birch
Copy Editor Cathy Lowne
Executive Art Editor Rozelle Bentheim
Designer Peter Gerrish
Picture Researchers Zoe Holtermann, Jennifer Veall
Production Controller Lucy Woodhead